Maidens by His Design

By Doran Richards

TEACHER'S GUIDE

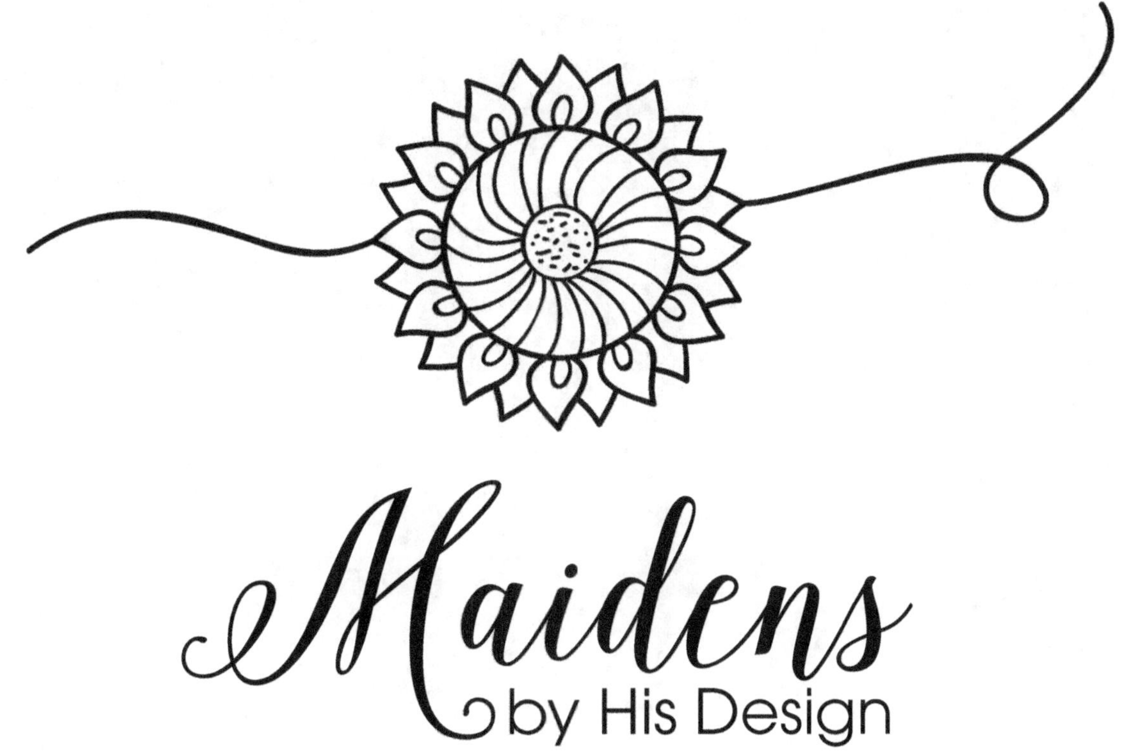

About Blessing God's Way

Blessing God's Way is a universal, international, non-denominational organization with the goal of implementing resources on maidenhood, maternity, and menopause within churches, communities, and other organizations that see the importance of proclaiming God as the Creator of women's life cycles.

Please visit **Blessing God's Way** at **www.BlessingGodsWay.com** for more information on how you can celebrate God's design for women!

Vision Statement
We desire to glorify God by honoring Him as Creator of the female body and to rejoice in His design for women in all seasons of life.

Mission Statement
The purpose of this ministry is to educate, edify, and celebrate God's special plan for women through maidenhood, maternity, and menopause.

Join Us
If you would like to join us in our efforts to spread this message far and wide, please join our Facebook page or email us to join the newsletter list.

Table of Contents

Introduction

Thank you for choosing to teach this course on how maidenhood is a blessing! Your desire to teach God as the Creator of this cycle in a young girl's life is an important step for her future cycles of pregnancy and menopause. This is an important first step in a life-long journey to see God's design for women.

In my desire to teach families about the blessings of pregnancy and childbearing, I realized something very important: that when teaching women about trusting in the process of childbearing (*i.e.*, taking responsibility for birth and erasing the spirit of fear), all of these things could be taught to young ladies about menses and menstruation as well. He created us and He created our cycles, thus we should look upon them as blessings, not curses.

I have designed this course for young ladies and their mothers (or aunts, grandmothers, and other women in the community) to learn about menstruation from a Biblical perspective. Just as with pregnancy and menopause, our daughters get bombarded with a negative worldview concerning their cycles, and I want to change that—with your help. This means reaching these young ladies *before* they are indoctrinated by the negative ideas of what it means to be a woman. To do this, we must bring God's name back into the center of all areas of women's lives, including menstruation.

Becoming a maturing maiden is a special time. It is an amazing process; so intricate that only God could have created it! We have to be careful when teaching this course, however. This is a process we should learn and trust, but we are not to worship it like some other faiths and cultures do. We worship God alone, He who created the process and He who created us. He is the Designer of our body and all of its processes.

As believers, we should rejoice and be content with the bodies given to us by God. As more young ladies are educated about the processes of their bodies, they come to trust it as a good design and take the fears surrounding it captive. We will then have well-supported young ladies who are confident with their bodies. This will lead to better birthing and menopausal stages of womanhood down the road because these young ladies are prepared for their life cycles from an early age. What a way to equip the next generation!

I hope this booklet and course will enable you to see maidenhood in a different, glorious light. It is time we reform our culture's views on maidenhood and menstruation!

Doran Richards - Founder, Blessing God's Way

Teaching This Course

This manual is composed of definitions, diagrams, and information taken from various sources which you will find in the **Works Cited** section at the end of this book. The scripture used in this text is from *The Message* version of the Bible by Eugene H. Peterson, unless otherwise indicated. I encourage you to use whatever version of the Bible you prefer. I chose this version because I believe that it speaks to the girls in language that they will easily understand and enjoy as they learn about their bodies.

This manual prepares you for each class and walks you through it step by step. The course is divided into chapters which can be taught one or more per week, depending on your time allowance; you could even teach the entire class in one weekend if you prefer. Each class is estimated to take about an hour, and the course is designed so that you can alter it to your timeframe.

A note on content: Chapter 9 of this Teacher's Guide covers numerous issues and abnormalities that can be part of the menstrual cycle, please use it at your own discretion. You may choose to copy the chapter to give to mothers for further research on menses, which will allow each mother to decide what to teach her daughter. Encourage mothers to be involved and to carefully screen what their daughters are learning.

This class is intended for girls between the ages of 8 to 15. Some girls may have already started their cycle but have not learned the terminology, or had opportunity to ask questions. Even if they have experienced what is being discussed, this course may give them a new perspective. The younger girls will be introduced to a lot of new information, so it is advisable to go slower for the younger ones and make sure they are able to follow along with the material. Younger girls will need the definitions to be as clear and simple as possible. Encourage older girls to speak and teach, which teaches young women to mentor their younger peers.

I advise that you make your sessions as interactive as possible to keep the young ladies engaged. To help them keep their focus, you will need to be creative and create games or fun ways of introducing the material as you go along. Drive home that this is a God-given design and they can be content and rejoice in it and get support from those around them. As the designer of this course, I encourage you to add your own personality and style to what is offered here. Each instructor will have a different gift to offer and will greatly enhance this program with that gift. What I have set before you is a basic outline and materials that cover the topics week by week.

Setting Up the Workshop

Thank you for responding to the call to bring *Maidens by His Design* to your local neighborhood! You need no special skills or training to teach this course; all adult woman are equipped to present it. It is a privilege to impact the future generations of women through the young girls and mothers you will be teaching. We hope that women and girls will come out of this course with a positive attitude about their bodies and confidence in the knowledge of how they were created. Please let us know when you plan to host your local *Maiden's by His Design* course so that we can help you advertise on the **Blessing God's Way** website and we can pray for you as you teach the class.

Deciding on a Timeline

Teaching this class is very flexible. It can completely fit your schedule, no matter the nature of the group you are teaching. The teaching timeline simply depends on availability of location and your preference. Some options to consider:

> **3 Week Series Class** - Three hour classes covering a chapter per hour with breaks at each hour.
>
> **5 Week Series Class** - Five classes of two hours each over a 5 week period. Cover two chapters per class.
>
> **10 Week Series Class** – Ten classes of one hour each over a 10 week period. This is good for homeschool groups, churches, girl scouts, or other organizations that may already meet on a similar schedule.

Location

The location can be your home, a friend's home, a local church, a local school, a library, etc. It should be a place that is convenient to both you and your class. Of course, the most important thing is to ensure the facility you choose will accommodate the number of students and parents you intend to register, so use your best judgment for location size.

Registering Students

Once you factor in your young students, their mothers/guardians, and other adults you may be teaching with, you will find that a class can get large rather quickly, so it is a good idea to allow no more than 16 girls to register for the class at a time. The nature of the course lends itself more readily to a smaller, more intimate group, which allows students to feel more comfortable and more inclined to open up more during discussion.

You may want to wait to see how many people register for the class before you order your workbooks. If you do not receive enough registering students to have a class, reconsider your marketing plan and reschedule the class for a future date. We can put your registration information on our website to help you advertise!

Collecting Payments and Registration Fees

It is up to you to set the price for your workshop registration fees. We recommend an amount of $85 per pair or mother/daughter team. Additional daughters/students could be asked to pay $60. Your expenses include: the teacher's guide, workbooks, materials for crafts, herbal samples, location fees, technology used to show video clips, resources to take and print a group photo, obtaining samples of personal care items for demonstrations and samples to handout, if desired, and creating fliers, if desired. As you can see, the girls are getting a real bargain! Anything you have left over can be used at your discretion.

Advertising

There are many ways of advertising your *Maiden's by His Design* workshop. Word of mouth is always a great tool to use! Encourage women to tell other women about this class throughout your community; tell a few people who you feel would be excited enough to tell others about it. Create flyers and post them in churches, daycares, libraries, schools, Christian businesses, health food stores—anywhere that you are able to post flyers and have them seen.

Make sure your event is easy to find online. Use social media to your advantage and include your event on Twitter, Facebook, Pinterest, Instagram, Yahoo Groups, Meetup, LinkedIn, Craigslist, or any other services you like to use. Send emails to friends, groups, schools, churches, and other acquaintances to spread the word about the upcoming class. You can even create your own event page on Facebook especially for your workshop. Let us know and we will link you to our **Maidens Facebook Page** as well!

Make sure that your class is posted on the **Blessing God's Way** website calendar. If not, send details about your class to info@blessinggodsway.com. We have a variety of marketing resources available to help you in your advertising efforts, including a song you can use, testimonials, frequently asked questions, and a sample outline of the class schedule. Contact us by email to have these files sent to you.

When you are advertising your workshop, please always reference that this curriculum is a **Blessing God's Way** curriculum and site our website as a reference.

Materials and Projects

Charting Resources

Having samples or information about different types of charting might be nice to show the mother/daughter teams. Some books are not entirely safe for young eyes, so having two stacks—one for moms and one for younger students—to use as samples might be helpful.

Herbal Products

You will need to purchase teas or herbal remedy products for use as samples in **Chapter 7**. We recommend visiting your local health food store to see if they can provide samples. Or you can create your own samples by purchasing small amounts and packaging them in small bags. You can also order anything you need online. For example, one company we have used online is Mountain Rose Herbs, though there are many others as well. This is an especially good idea If you intend to teach more than one class. If you are unable to find samples, you may simply have pictures of different herbs taken from websites, books, or magazines. You may be able to find books on herbs from your local library for reference.

I like to prepare some **NORA tea** beforehand and take it with me to allow the girls to sample at the event. You will need a pitcher and disposable cups if you choose to do this. NORA stands for Nettles, Oatstraw, Red Raspberry Leaf, and Alfalfa. This will be a loose-leaf tea. Order each of the separate herbs online or buy from your local source and then combine in the following proportions:

- 2 parts Red Raspberry Leaf
- 2 parts Nettles
- 1 part Oatstraw
- 1 part Alfalfa

To brew the tea:

- Boil water in tea kettle or pot, using a thick glass vessel such as a canning jar.
- Add approx. 2 inches of mixed herbs to the bottom of the jar and then pour hot water on top.
- Mix well, cover with lid, and allow to steep for several hours or overnight.
- Strain herbs out with a fine mesh sieve or clean cloth, carefully saving the tea in your serving pitcher.
- Sweeten to taste with stevia, coconut sugar, or turbinado sugar, as you desire. You can also add fresh lemon juice if you like.

It can be served hot or cold. Don't forget to bring paper cups to pass out samples at your event. I recommend that women drink this tea in all seasons of their lives since it has multiple benefits. It is especially helpful to boost iron levels, stabilize hormones, and ease cramps during the menstruation phase of your cycle.

(I like to sweeten the tea with organic coconut sugar, stevia, or honey but do not make it too sweet so they can taste the herbs in the final tea blend.)

NOTE: You will also find this recipe for NORA tea in **Chapter 7**, where we will discuss the ingredients and their beneficial properties in more depth.

Samples and "Goody Bags"

It is nice to have some samples of various tools and gear to demonstrate to the girls. Explain that the girls may wish to have something on hand when they show signs of womanhood, so they are prepared when they start their cycle.

Examples of pads, pantyliners, tampons, menstrual cups, cloth pads, and bras for young ladies are all nice to have. These should be clean and unused. You may wish to explain the health benefits of natural and breathable fabrics and materials for these items.

You can order these items online, buy in stores, or contact companies and request samples for your maidenhood workshop. Some companies we have worked with include:

- Natracare
- Lifegiving Linen
- Kotex Natural Balance
- Yellowberry Bras
- Diva Cup
- La Luna Cup
- Floradix
- Softcup
- Party in my Pants Pads
- Glad Rags

Lapbook Projects

The lapbook projects are a fun way for the girls to create something tangible from what they are learning in this course. You are free to provide any materials for them to use with their projects—get creative! You can purchase supplies yourself from craft stores, dollar stores, or online stores; you can include this cost in the registration fee or charge a fee for supplies. Alternatively, you may tell your students to each bring in a donation of craft supplies to share with everyone.

Suggested materials include: printed scriptures, quotes from the workbooks or other uplifting sources, Christian stickers, yarn or ribbon for making borders, colored paper, beads or glitter, etc. You will need glue, scissors, pens/markers, and other basic craft tools. Pre-cut all the papers into workable sizes and pre-package everything into individual bags. Having a kit with blank booklet, papers, glue sticks, and pictures ready to go will make passing out the supplies easy and organized. Have markers or colored pens available for girls to write with as well.

Don't forget to include a photograph of your class in the craft kit so the girls can glue it in their lapbook project and remember the friends they made during the workshop. You will need to plan a way to take and print the photo in advance. (One idea is to take the photo with a disposable camera at the beginning of class and run to a photo printing center during the lunch hour to get the images developed. Another way is to bring a digital camera and photo printer with you to the workshop or ask your facility if a color printer is available. If you use a digital camera or your cell phone camera, you can upload your image to a photo printing center such as Walmart or Walgreens using a cell phone app or website and then pick up the prints the same day.) Make sure you plan ahead and test that the technology you choose will work the day of your event.

You can find more information and instructions for this project in **Chapter 10**.

Tips for Teaching

Introduce yourself and explain why you are teaching the course. Start the workshop off with a fun icebreaker activity. One example: have each girl randomly select a colored bead. Each color will correlate with a pre-chosen question that the girl must answer about herself. For instance, if the girl chooses a green bead she must name her favorite food, or if she chooses a red bead she must name the last book she read. Have this written down beforehand so you remember.

Take some group photos at the beginning of the class for their craft activity, both a serious picture and a silly one. Include the moms in the photo, too. Select the best image and make a plan to print the photos so each girl has one to keep.

Try to make teaching the event as fun and engaging as possible. Depending on the age of the girls, attention spans can be limited. Notify the parents in advance that they should explain to their girls that the workshop is both educational *and* fun.

When you explain the "gear and tools" portion of the course (**Chapter 2**), gather the girls around you so everyone can see the samples that you brought. Allow the girls to touch and ask questions about what they see.

Encourage a safe, intimate atmosphere for asking questions. I like to have girls write down anonymous questions on notecards and collect them so I can then provide the answers or have the other mothers give answers. (You can do this towards the beginning or middle of the course.) This takes the pressure off the girls and helps prevent embarrassment. Encourage the young ladies to go to their parents with any questions or concerns they may have in the future as well.

Use the quizzes and games provided in the workbooks to your advantage and encourage participation from both moms and girls. I like to have moms competing against the girls in the games to create some fun competition. Each activity and quiz in this Teacher's Guide has the page number for the Student Workbook listed for your easy reference while teaching.

I also make a point to have the mothers share their stories about entering into womanhood; you may start by sharing your own story and then opening up the floor for anyone that would like to share something. Story sharing is discussed in **Chapter 6**.

You may choose to include a closing prayer in your teaching, if you feel it is appropriate.

Also, don't forget to take breaks and give the girls a chance to stretch periodically.

Hand out certificates at the end of your workshop and congratulate each girl on completing the *Maidens by His Design* course!

Evaluation Forms

In the **Appendix** of your teacher's guide is a sample evaluation form you can copy if you would like. We also have a PDF version available online. You can pass out this optional form if you would like to receive feedback on your teaching at the end of your course.

Thank-you for choosing to teach a *Maidens by His Design* course in your neighborhood! It blesses our ministry and warms our hearts to know that seeds of knowledge are being planted in the minds of young girls near and far. It will bless the lives of each girl you reach as they learn and understand God's glorious design for their bodies.

Acknowledgements

The very first "thank you" must go to God! Almighty God has to be praised and thanked for putting this project on my heart. It was an overwhelming "voice," to say the least. I have only tried to be obedient to that voice. I feel blessed and honored to be used for His service in this way

The process of compiling information for this book was a team effort. What you have before you has only come into being from the most dedicated and diligent work of so many wonderful ladies on the **Blessing God's Way** team.

Special thanks and gracious gratitude goes to all the wonderful souls over the last 18 years who have worked passionately on this project with me. Some of these women have been with me through thick and thin, and are not only loyal, but trustworthy and humble: Rachel Himelright for partnering with me to create the My Personal Proverbs section, Emma Potter, my daughter, who has been with me since the beginning and took this course at its birth and completion while looking over my should while it was being created, Michele Wheaton for contributing and never losing interest in this material and what it teaches, Amber Troska who stepped up to help me with the beginning of the expansion and updating while offering lovely editing skills, Exodus Design for finishing this life-long dream of mine to have it complete and offered worldwide to women and daughters everywhere. Special thanks to my family for supporting and encouraging me along this very mountainous terrain, and all the ups and downs that go with that journey.

Materials List

Chapter One:

>Camera for taking class photo
>
>Diagram of female body, enlarged (optional)
>
>Beads for the icebreaker activity (optional)

Chapter Two:

>Samples of pads, and other menstrual supplies

Chapter Three:

>N/A

Chapter Four:

    Treats/prizes for game

    Index cards for anonymous questions

Chapter Five:

    N/A

Chapter Six:

    Treats/prizes for game

Chapter Seven:

    NORA Tea Samples

    Gallon container / Disposable cups for tea

    Sweetener

Chapter Eight:

    N/A

Chapter Nine:

    Index cards or small slip of paper

    Blank diagram 2 for review

    Treat/prizes for passing quiz

Chapter Ten:

    File folders or plain white booklets for lapbooks

    Supplies for lapbooks (stickers, decorative paper, etc)

    Pens/pencils/markers

    Tape, glue, staplers

Chapter 1
WHAT IS MENSTRUATION?

This is the first day with your students—make it light and fun! Be sure to give the students and parents an opportunity to ask question along the way.

Always begin class with prayer and hand out the student workbooks. Explain that you will be collecting workbooks after each session (if teaching over 5-week or 10-week timeframe) to help keep them private and so they won't forget them at home for future gatherings. Students will take their workbooks home at the end of the course.

Consider introducing a couple of ice breakers at the start of class, allowing the students and moms to get to know each other a little more and to lighten the mood. These types of openers can be found by googling "ice breakers for parties," etc. Find one or two that seem appropriate for young ladies and use them however you think works best.

Beginning the Course

Introduction of the Teacher
Introduce yourself to the class. Tell them why you are passionate about this subject and why you have chosen to teach it. Give them some background as to why you would choose to bring this curriculum to this particular community of women.

Introduction of the Course
Tell the class about this program and some of the things they will learn; a simple overview of chapter titles is sufficient. Let them know they are going to have a great time and that all material covered in this class is to be **kept confidential**. Tell students that this subject matter is not something that ought to be shared freely with friends or other people without permission from their parents.

Have scriptures written on the board before class begins. The scriptures will also be included in the students' workbooks. They are scriptures that support teaching our daughters about this design—just like any other area of life. It is important to learn about purity, modesty, and Christian character, but it is also important to learn about our bodies and the way God designed them.

Why This Course?
When updating the curriculum, I was browsing through other books that talked about and taught about menstruation to girls and young women. I thought to myself, "there are so many other resources out there already, why am I making this update?" but as I continued my research, I realized that there isn't anything out there pointing our girls to the Creator of this design.

3 Reasons This Course and Curriculum Are Important (SW-pg1):

1. God's Design. This course is written to help women see menses and/or menstruation from a Biblical perspective. This is God's design and we should acknowledge it as such when teaching our daughters about this special time in their lives. He is the designer of the design of menstruation.

> **Romans 12:1-2 -** So here's what I want you to do, God helping you: Take your everyday, ordinary life - your sleeping, eating, going-to-work, and walking-around life - and place it before God as an offering. Embracing what God does for you is the best thing you can do for him. Don't become so well-adjusted to your culture that you fit into it without even thinking. Instead, fix your attention on God. You'll be changed from the inside out. Readily recognize what he wants from you, and quickly respond to it. Unlike the culture around you, always dragging you down to its level of immaturity, God brings the best out of you, develops well-formed maturity in you.

> **Job 10:8 -** You made me like a handcrafted piece of pottery—and now are you going to smash me to pieces? Don't you remember how beautifully you worked my clay? Will you reduce me now to mud pie?

2. Conquering Fear. There is a need for this information because our daughters are scared and anxious when it comes to this time in their lives and God tells us not to have a spirit of fear. This course is important because God tells us to get wisdom; learning is important to Him.

> **II Timothy 1:7 -** God doesn't want us to be shy with his gifts, but bold and loving and sensible.

> **Proverbs 2:10-11 -** Lady Wisdom will be your close friend, and Brother Knowledge your pleasant companion. Good Sense will scout ahead for danger, Insight will keep an eye out for you.

> **Proverbs 4:3-7 -** Sell everything and buy Wisdom! Forage for Understanding! Don't forget one word! Don't deviate an inch!

3. Holistic Health. There are so many other issues surrounding the changes that attend puberty in girls. It is not just a physical event, but a holistic event encompassing mind, body and spirit.

> **1 Corinthians 15:44 -** Put in the ground weak, it comes up powerful. The seed sown is natural; the seed grown is supernatural—same seed, same body, but what a difference from when it goes down in physical mortality to when it is raised up in spiritual immortality!

> **3 John 1:2 -** How I truly love you! We're the best of friends, and I pray for good fortune in everything you do, and for your good health—that your everyday affairs prosper, as well as your soul!

Basic Body Design (SW-pg 2)

Now we need to go over some definitions and basic bodily functions. We will label the body parts that are affected by our menstrual cycle to better familiarize ourselves with how we as women are designed by God.

Getting as many facts as we can will enable us to trust the process of menstruation and help us to not to be anxious about this cycle in our lives. This will also prepare us for the other cycles we will face as women: maternity and menopause. God tells us to get wisdom and understanding—let us begin to do so!

Basic Definitions
Here are some basic definitions of terms we will be using. **NOTE: Students will have blank diagrams (SW-pg3) in their workbooks to fill out in CHAPTER 1.**

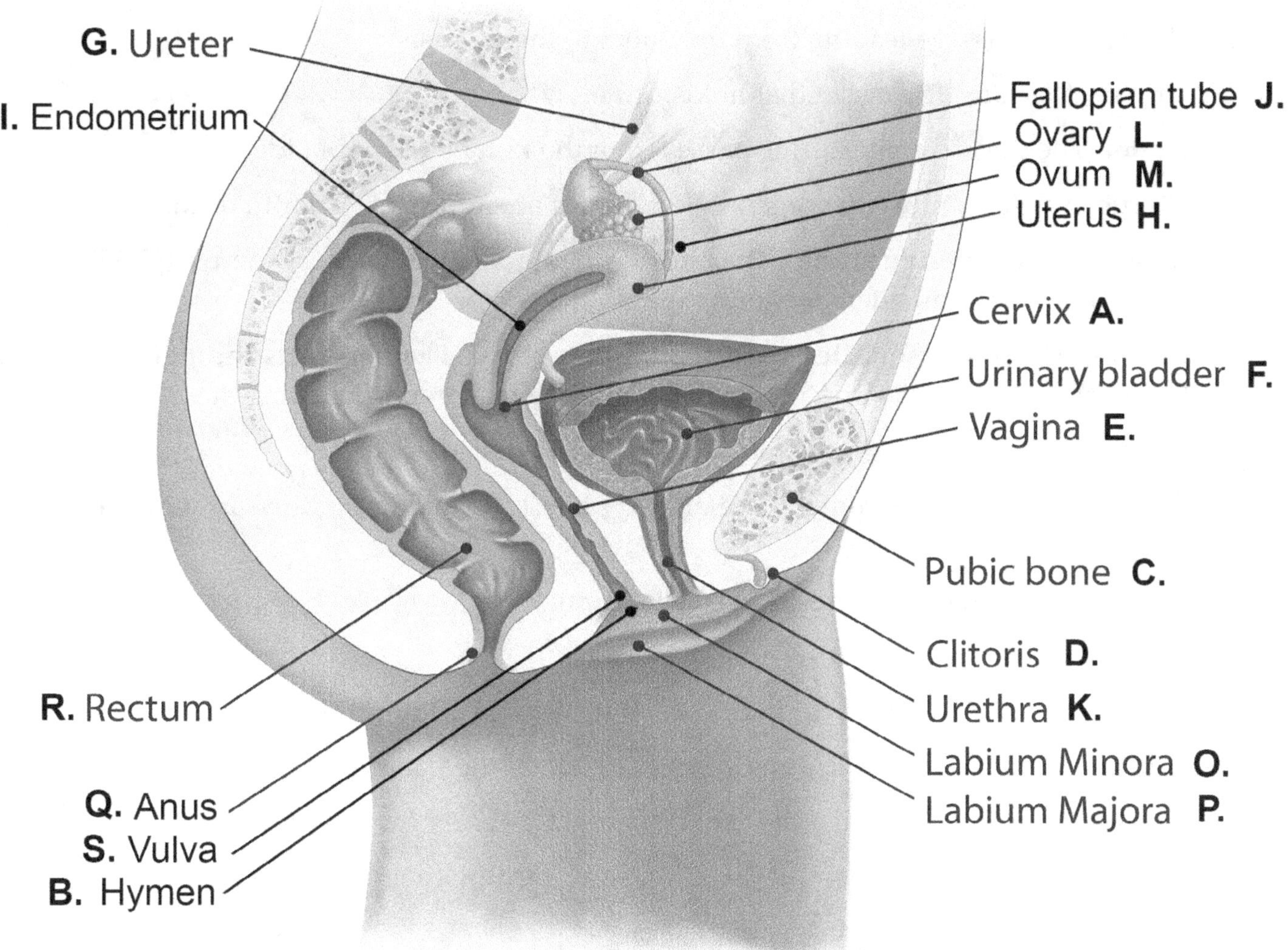

Diagram 1.1 – The Female Reproductive System - Side Body View

Explain to the students that this is the basic terminology, and while they may not understand all the terms yet, they will by the end of the course. Also explain that they will see these terms quite a bit throughout the course. Go over each part and briefly discuss its location (definitions below). **Have the students fill out the blanks (SW-pg 4) in their workbooks.** Ask if anyone knows about these parts already, and how they learned about them.

A. **Cervix:** A circular structure at the bottom of the uterus and at the top of the vaginal wall that opens and stretches.

B. **Hymen**: A thin membrane partly closing the external vaginal opening.

C. **Pubic Bone**: The bone that sits on top of your bladder.

D. **Clitoris**: A small, sensitive part of the female genitals at the anterior (upper) end of the vulva.

E. **Vagina**: The passage leading from the vulva to the uterus.

F. **Urinary Bladder**: The organ that holds urine.

G. **Ureter**: The duct by which urine passes from the kidney to the bladder.

H. **Uterus**: A hollow, muscular organ where babies are nourished prior to birth.

I. **Endometrium (uterine lining)**: The mucous membrane that lines the uterus. (**NOTE:** Point to the uterus to show them the lining)

J. **Fallopian Tubes (also called oviducts)**: Either of two slender ducts through which ova (eggs) pass from the ovaries to the uterus in the female reproductive system.

K. **Urethra**: Where urine travels from the bladder to outside of body.

L. **Ovary**: The female reproductive gland, typically occurring in pairs, in which eggs are produced.

M. **Ovum (Egg)**: A female reproductive cell. Plural: Ova.

N. **Ovulate**: To produce and discharge ova.

O. **Labium Minora**: Tissue surrounding the outside area of the vagina opening.

P. **Labium Majora**: Tissue surrounding the outside of the Labium Minora.

Q. **Anus**: Opening at the end of the canal where we get rid of waste (bowels).

R. **Rectum**: The final section of the large intestine, terminating at the anus.

S. **Vulva:** Opening of the vaginal canal.

NOTE: Did you know that it wasn't until 1863 that they discovered that we had ovaries and ovum? Science is always changing and discovering new things, including how our bodies work from the inside out.

Refer students to **Diagram 1.2** (SW-pg 5) in their workbooks. Point out that this is the "frontal view" of **Diagram 1.1** and contains the same parts. Take a few moments to let them look at it, study it, and discuss it. Have the students fill in each blank in their workbook as you discuss it. It is helpful if you hold up one of the diagrams to the student's body, showing them where that would be (it is a nice visual for them and they often find it funny). You can enlarge and print or project the diagrams and use that as a visual as you teach as well.

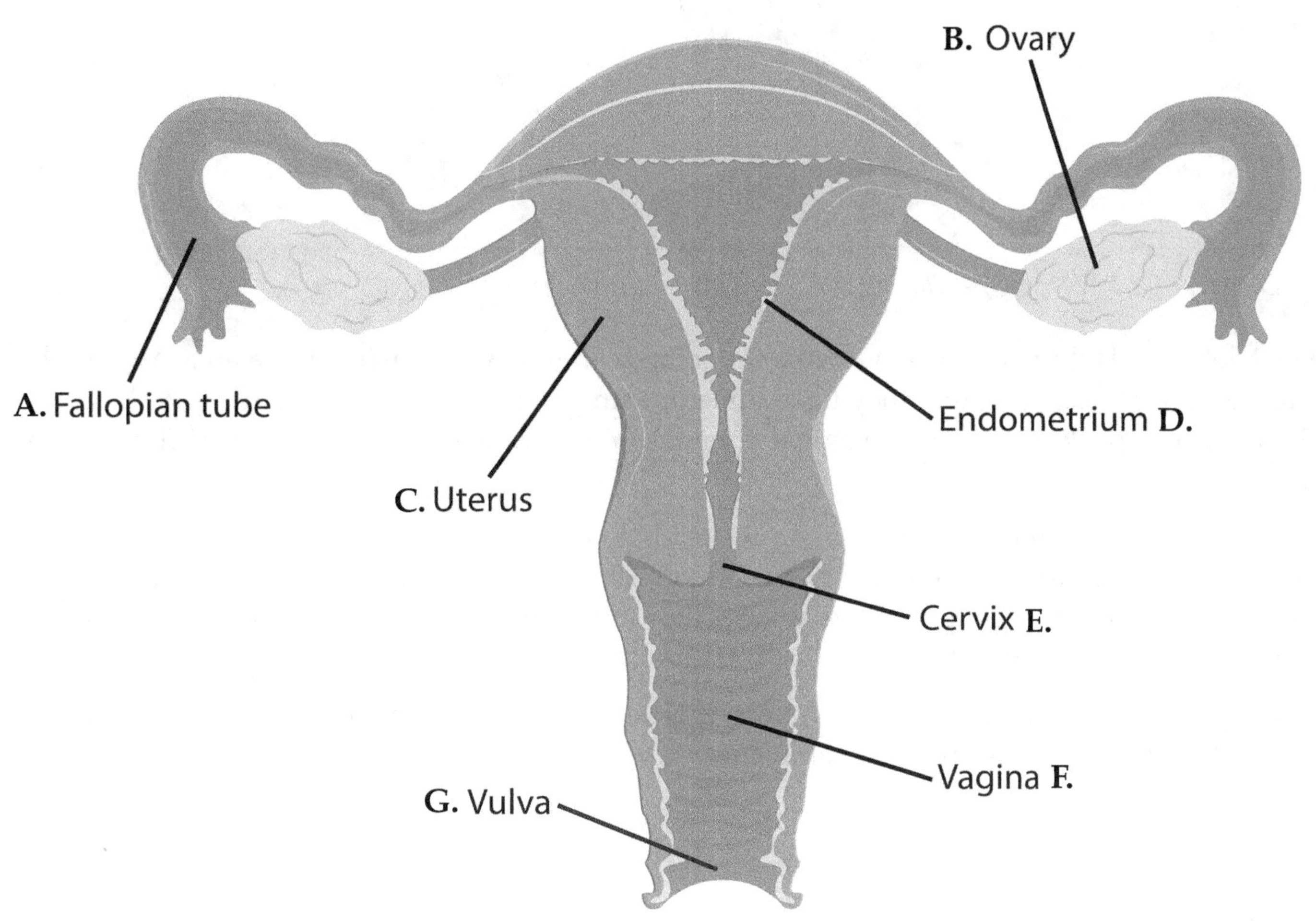

Diagram 1.2 – The Female Reproductive System - Front View

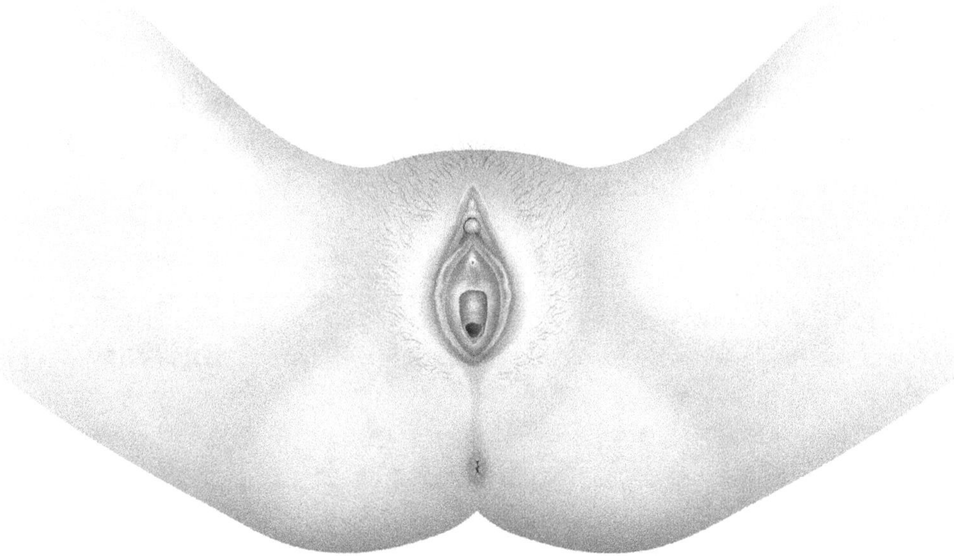

Diagram 1.3 (SW-pg 6) – The Female Anatomy - Bottom View

NOTE: A lot of girls do not realize how many openings they have in their private area. You might want to point out to the girls that they have three openings: the **urethra**, the **vagina**, and the **anus**. Tell them we are speaking about the vaginal opening in this course; that is where their flow comes from.

Showing the girls different angles of their bodies helps them understand the placement of the different parts being introduced in this class. Don't rush through this part—it is important for the rest of the course that they get familiar with how they are created and the names of those parts that make up the body designed for them.

Now we will talk a little about the actual monthly cycle. Tell the ladies to please follow along and to stop you if they have any questions or comments.

Menstrual Cycle

Your cycle begins on the first day of your discharge, or menstrual flow, and lasts until the next first day of your flow, when the cycle begins again. Some women consider the menstrual cycle to be only the bleeding time itself, but the cycle actually consists of the whole process our bodies go through each month, including non-bleeding days.

In this awesome and fascinating cycle, our bodies are releasing eggs from our ovaries (the ovaries take turns each month) as well as preparing our uterine lining, which is called the **endometrium**, for a pregnancy. If the egg is not fertilized*, causing pregnancy, the lining of our uterus must be shed. The word menstruation is used for the **first day** of your bleeding, not the whole cycle. (***NOTE:** Fertilization means the egg has met with sperm and created a pregnancy. Each mother can explain more of this particular process to her daughter when she feels the time is right to do so.)

Menstrual Cycle Length & Phases (SW-pg 7)

Your cycle may vary in its length. An average cycle is 29.5 days but can be as much as 35 days from start to finish. The number of days will vary from one woman to another. Note that young ladies just beginning their cycle may experience irregularity for the first year or so. This is normal.

The cycle is broken up into four phases. These phases will help you see what your body is doing and why. **NOTE:** This diagram can be written on the board or otherwise shared for them to see how it is a true cycle.

There are four stages of our menstrual cycle:

- **Menstruation**
- **Follicular**
- **Ovulation**
- **Luteal**

NOTE: These monthly cycles last about 40 years in our womanhood, ending at menopause, when our cycle begins to become less regular and then cease altogether. Mentioning this will give the girls a chance to see the big picture of menstruating and that it doesn't last their entire lifetime.

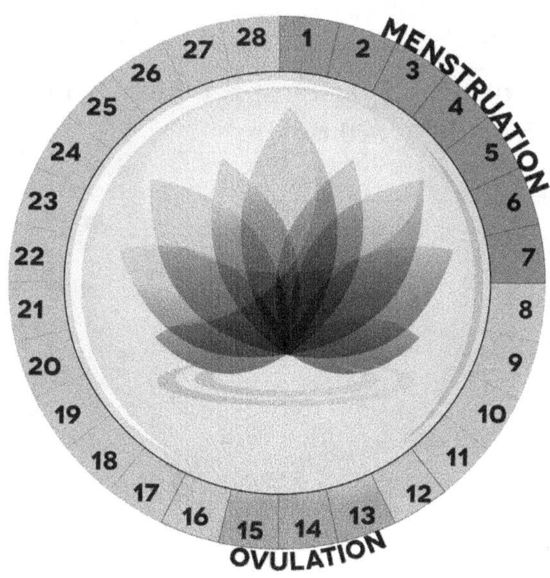

Diagram 1.4 - Menstrual Phases

MENSTRUATION: *Menstruation* occurs when the broken-down lining of the uterus flows out through the vagina. This is called your "period," or "flow." Menstrual flow may last anywhere from 3-7 days. The length will vary and may not be regular when you first begin your period or for the first year or so of cycling.

FOLLICULAR: The *follicular phase* is the phase when a follicle (a sac that contains an egg) in the ovary develops and matures. Only one ovary each month will produce a follicle. The developing follicle produces the female hormone **estrogen** which causes the lining of the uterus (**endometrium**) to become build up or thicken in preparation for a pregnancy. (Remind them where the lining is located inside the uterus.)

OVULATION: *Ovulation* occurs when the mature egg is expelled (or bursts) from its follicle. Ovulation happens on about day 14 (two weeks after your cycle started) of an average 28-day menstrual cycle. This phase takes 24-48 hours to complete and is the shortest phase.

LUTEAL: The *luteal phase* is the time from ovulation (on about day 14) to the beginning of menstruation.

The menstrual cycle doesn't have to be a "drag" or "curse." Our culture often sees it in a negative light, but it actually shows how complex your body is and is a sign that your body is functioning properly. God is so good! *(We will talk more about your phases in this course when teaching about charting your cycle in Chapter 4.)*

High levels of hormones are working inside your body throughout your cycle—all in preparation for an egg to either implant in your uterus or to be expelled with your period. *(We talk in depth about hormones in Chapter 4 as well.)*

Students have blank lines to list the four phases of the menstrual cycle (SW-pg 8) **in the Student Workbook. Give them time to write the word down.**

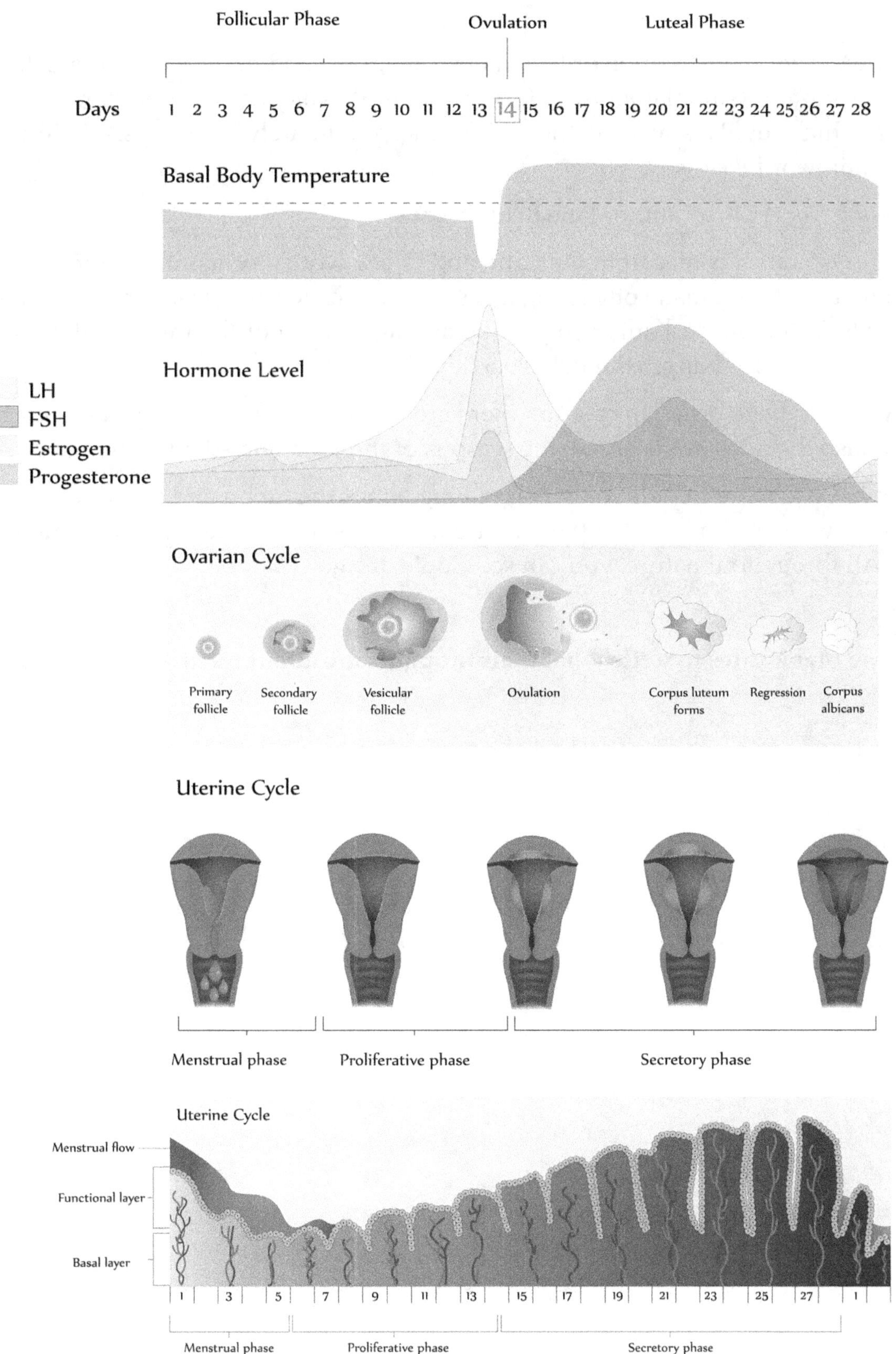

Diagram 1.5 - Whole Body Cycle in Phases (SW-pg 9)

Menses (SW-pg10)

Menses is another word for menstruation or the "menstrual flow" and derives from the Latin word *menses*, which means months (singular *mensis* refers to 1 month). Note that the word "moon,"—as in the Earth's moon, which revolves around the Earth in approximately 29.5 days,—is likewise is derived from the Latin word *mensis*.

In the book *A Blessing Not A Curse*, author Jane Bennett says:

> "The word *menstruation* comes from the Latin and Greek words for month and moon. *Mensis* means moon in Latin, and many other languages have words for menstruation that correspond to their words for moon. Not surprisingly, the average length of the menstrual cycle is the same as the lunar cycle at approximately 29.5 days."

God created the world to have order. In creation there are other areas that have cycles—our bodies and the moon, but also the tides in the ocean, the seasons of the year, and so much more.

NOTE: We do not have to have trepidation when talking about the moon and its cycle and how it relates to our cycle as women. God created the moon, stars, and sun, and He has also created us. He is a God of order. All throughout nature, you can see God's design.

Students have some blank lines to write what their thoughts are about mentruation or a monthly cycle (SW-p10).

Chapter 2
WE ARE FEARFULLY & WONDERFULLY MADE

REVIEW (SW-p11)

Review last week's definitions and ask for questions or comments in regards to what they have learned so far. Test them on some definitions by pointing to one of the diagrams from week one and see if they remember the terms.

Blood Talk

Here we will discuss the "blood" part of our menstruation with your class or workshop.

Menstruation is God's special plan for us as women. He has chosen to bless us with this gift because it enables us to bear children one day, LORD willing. Menstruation is experienced by all healthy women for most of their lives. Yet it is a topic cloaked in secrecy, taboo, and negativity. Few women see the positive side to this life cycle.

When girls are asked what they think of their period, most girls consider it an inconvenient nuisance, something dirty or disgusting. Only about 1% believe it is their body functioning normally! How sad that is. We, as Christian girls and women, can do better than that! We can glorify God by showing Him that we believe His process of menstruation is good!

Bring the student's attention to the questions section in the box in the student workbook. Go over these points with them. I like to have the students take turns reading them and answering them out loud.

ACTIVITY: Some Questions About Menstruation

Are you afraid to think of the blood coming out of your body during menstruation?
Most girls are. Learning about our cycle helps to eliminate an anxious mind. Trusting in God's design helps us feel comfortable with our bodies.

How much will you bleed?
Not as much as you think. On average, a few spoonfuls to a half-cup is shed each month. When you begin your cycle for the first time, bleeding or discharge will probably be minimal and very light. Once your cycle becomes more regular, it will increase somewhat.

How many days will you bleed?
It varies between individuals, but usually anywhere from 3-7 days. It can start out light, then have a day or so of heavier discharge before becoming light again. It can be the reverse, beginning heavy and becoming lighter, or be about the same throughout the menstruation period.

Is Menstruation "Unclean"? (SW-p12)

Let's see how scripture talks about the blood. Some biblical descriptions of what it signifies might help us see that this is a wonderful process, created by a loving God and Father.

The main references are the ones in Leviticus that explain the unclean laws that require separation for a period of time during the days of a woman's cycle. God has a purpose for this. This doesn't mean that women or young ladies are dirty or disgusting. It merely means that they are having fluid come from them, making them unclean for a period of time (3 to 7 days). We can trust in God's purpose for having a period of separation.

> **Leviticus 15:19:** When a woman has a discharge of blood, the impurity of her menstrual period lasts seven days. Anyone who touches her is unclean until evening. Everything on which she lies or sits during her period is unclean. Anyone who touches her bed or anything on which she sits must wash his clothes and bathe in water; he remains unclean until evening.

This is saying that she has discharge, nothing more, nothing less. She is reported to be unclean, but that is only because a fluid is leaking from her body during menstruation.

Blood has a significant importance in our lives—we cannot ignore this fact. Blood is cleansing to us when it is talked about in the Bible. Blood was shed for us; it cleanses us and protects us from sin. Only the LORD could make such a substance clean us. Our monthly blood, mixed with cells and tissue, cleanses our insides to prepare for a new cycle, just as Jesus' blood cleanses us from sin. Isn't that fascinating? How awesome is our God?

Ask the class, "What else can you think uses blood to cleanse?" they have blank lines in their book to write (answer: wounds, having a baby, menopause)

NOTE: Please know that we are not comparing Jesus' blood to our monthly blood in any way that suggests they are equal, but blood often represents cleansing in the Bible. Even in the Old Testament, blood had to be shed to cleanse people from their sins.

Gear for Our Cycle (SW-p13)

Let us look at some tools or "gear" that will help us through our menstruating time. **(NOTE: Have some samples of different sized pads, panty liners, wings and tampons for the students to see.)** Show them a cloth pad, a "keeper" or menstrual cup, and sponges as alternatives to disposable products, if you have them. Explain that reusable products help save the environment and are healthier in general. Also mention how we want to use products on our bodies, and our sensitive tissue down there, that is as free of chemicals as possible.

Here are examples of gear for our menstrual cycle:

PADS

There are a few different types of sanitary napkins or pads to use during your cycle. When you start your menstruation for the first time, you may only need light panty liners. You might want to use the longer, thicker ones for night time, which will help you not leak blood / fluid on your clothes and bed. During the end of your period, you might want to simply use the light day pads that are very thin and small, which are ideal for catching that last day or so of discharge.

Be aware that there are alternatives to disposable sanitary pads or napkins as well. They are called Glad Rags, Luna Pads (brand names), or just cotton pads. These can be a great alternative because they are organic and gentler on your skin. Store-bought products can be bleached and contain chemicals that could be an irritant or cause health problems. These also are reusable and do not take up space as trash in landfills.

If students feel uncomfortable with the idea of reusable pads, please share this from the Glad Rags website:

> "Reusable pads. That's gross!" That's a comment we've heard and one we might have made ourselves before we really thought about it. But just envision your lifetime supply of used pads and tampons in landfills or washed up on a beach. Now that's gross!"

TAMPONS

Tampons are slender, tube-shaped products that are usually made of cotton. They are inserted inside your body (vagina) and absorb the fluid as it flows out. Keep in mind that there is a potential **health hazard** (toxic shock syndrome) that can come from wearing disposable tampons for too long, so be sure to go over this with your mother and read the inserts that come in the box. There are natural alternatives to tampons, called sponges, that you can use in place of a disposable tampon.

NATURAL SPONGES

You can purchase actual natural sponges shaped like a tampon to use a more natural product compared to the store-bought, bleached tampons that are most common.

MENSTRUAL CUPS AND KEEPERS

Menstrual cups are products often known under brand names like "The Diva Cup" or "The Keeper," that women can use as an alternative to a tampon or pad. Some are latex and some are not and they are inserted into the body, similar to a tampon or sponge. They are reusable rather than disposable and don't have any harmful chemicals in them. If you opt for a menstrual cup, you rinse it out instead of changing it for a new one and they come in different sizes. Many companies sell these, including Lena, Athena, Vida, and others, so do the research and find a company you want to support.

NOTE: explain to your students that the samples you have might be for women older than they are, who have had children before, etc. These companies make small sizes for girls just beginning their cycle.

REVIEW

Discuss the hygiene "gear" options available to them that can be purchased from the store as well as ordered online or made at home. Be clear about which ones are environmentally good choices and why some are not. Find out what products they might prefer and what feelings and opinions led them prefer some choices over others and why that might be.

To conclude this chapter with a positive thought, you have the option to read this little excerpt from the Glad Rags website (www.gladrags.com), or you can highlight sentences that you would like your audience to hear:

Menstrual Musings (SW-p13)

"The menstrual cycle is a healthy and natural process. However, in our culture we have been led to believe it is a messy inconvenience to be kept secret, or worse, a repugnant disease-like condition. We encourage you to examine your beliefs about menstruation carefully. Any embarrassment or shame you may feel could be the result of culturally-inspired negative conditioning. How we perceive and interpret the feelings that accompany our cycles can have a dramatic effect on our health. Imagine the self-fulfilling destiny of the girl who hears, "Now you've got the curse, get ready for cramps, and a bloody mess.""

Want to make your own pad? Here are instructions!

These instructions are in the student workbook (SW-p14).

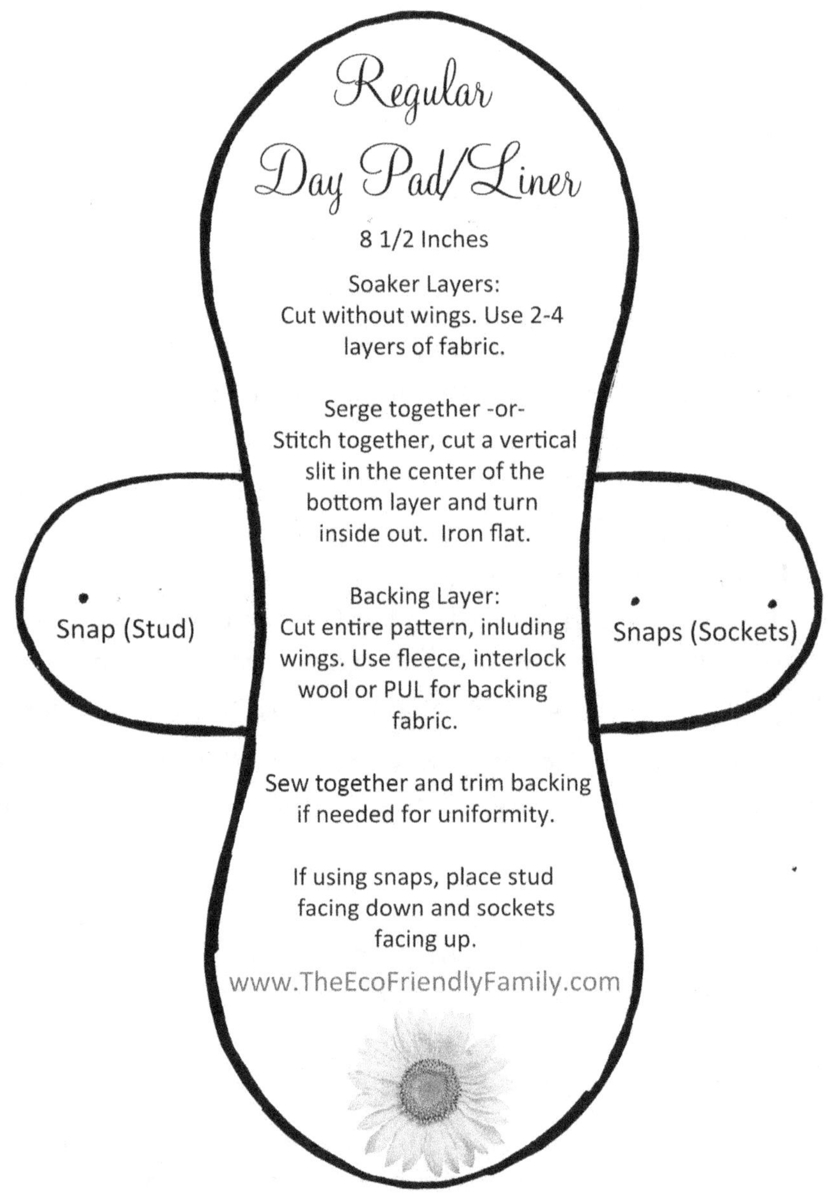

ACTIVITY: Name The Product: (SW-p15)

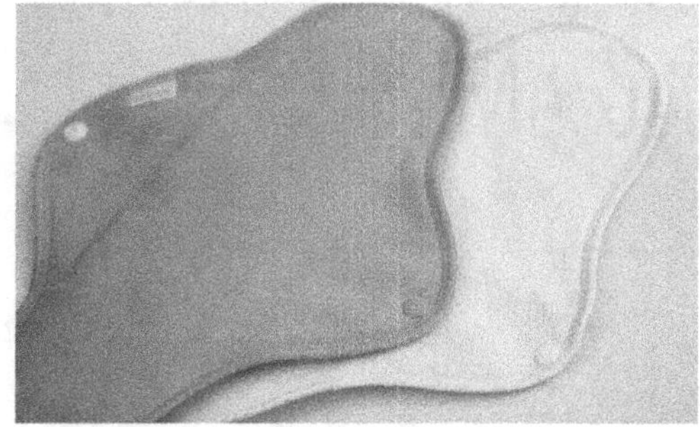

1. Glad Rags/Luna Pads

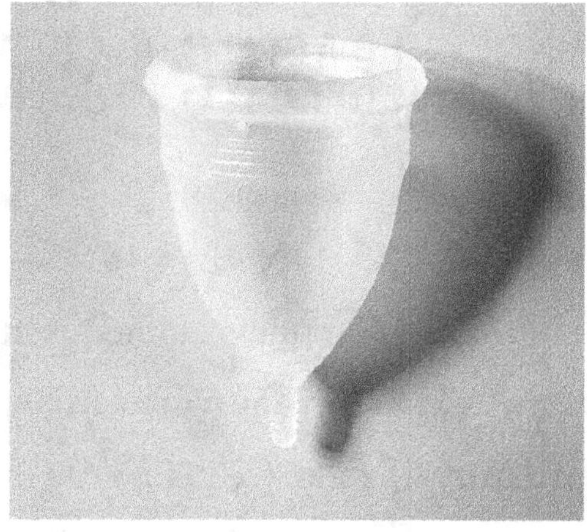

2. Menstrual Cup/Keeper

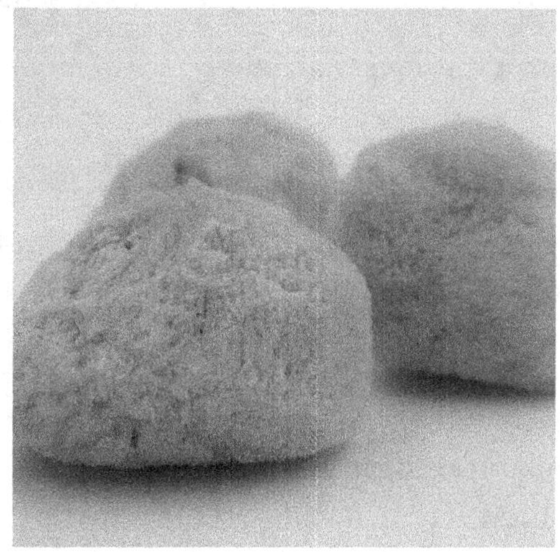

3. Natural Sponges

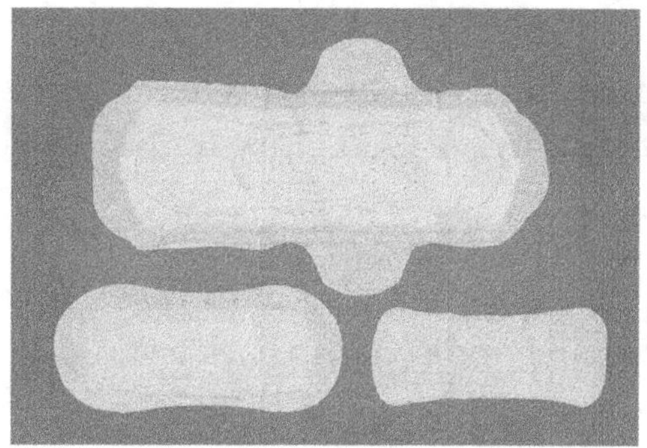

4. Disposable Pads & Liners

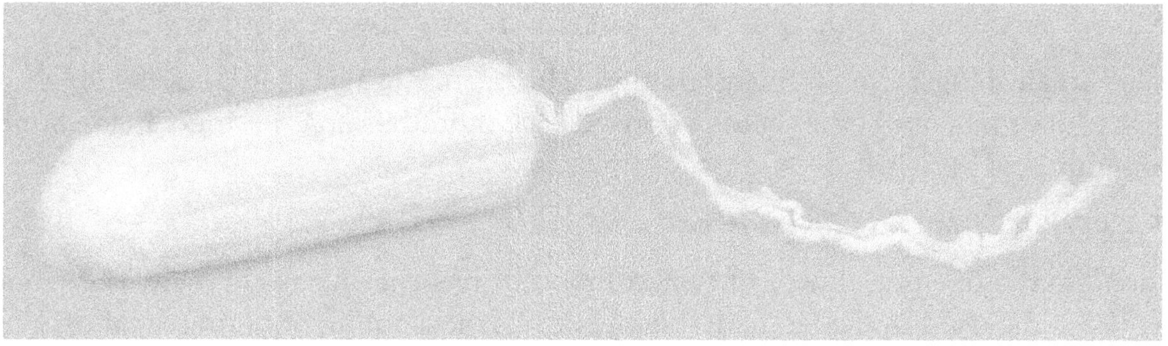

5. Tampons

Chapter 3
ERASING A SPIRIT OF FEAR & ANXIETY

REVIEW DISCUSSION (SW-p16)

- What products did their mother used when she started her period?

- What would they name a menstrual product and why?

The Definition of Fear (NOTE: write this definition on the board and use it for this discussion)

> *an unpleasant, often strong emotion caused by anticipation or awareness of danger; b: (1) an instance of this emotion; (2) state marked by the emotion.*
>
> *anxious concern.*

Not having a spirit of fear or not being anxious takes work—hard work—but with support and love we defeat it and give God glory for our cycle of menstruation!

Mabel Hale in *Beautiful Girlhood*, says:

> "Every day our girls will meet with circumstances in which she has her choice between frowning and sending back a stinging retort, or smiling and passing them by with a kind word. If she can pass these little bumps and keep sweet, then she has mastered the art of being sunny."

She also states:

> "Live in the sunshine. Look on the bright side, for there is always a bright side."

God is revealed in all things, even in menstruation. The beauty of His plan and His love for us is manifested in the design of our bodies being cleansed each month. He has lovingly made our bodies capable of being purged regularly.

Consider another quote from *Beautiful Girlhood*:

> "Girlhood is the opening flower of womanhood. It has charms all its own. The wonderful change from the child to the woman, the marvelous blossoming of young, healthy girlhood, will ever be God's great miracle in life's garden."

Reclaiming this time of our lives, showing God's good and great design, is yet one more way we as Christians can be a shining lights in a negative culture; one more way we can show God's grace, mercy, and majesty. Our daughters can be set apart in this area——apart from the secular world— giving God the glory, honor, and praise for such a gift as this. You do not do this in a public square, announcing it from the rooftops, but you can show contentedness and joy even during your cycle. We are His workmanship.

Genesis 1:31 God looked over everything he had made; it was so good, so very good! (SW-p17)

ACTIVITY: Share your fears

Have your students write a fear or anxiety they might have in regards to maturing, the processes of menstruation, or what to expect during their cycle. Hand out small slips of paper or index cards and let them know they do not have to put their names on them. It is anonymous and they can feel safe opening up and asking what might be on their mind at this point in the learning process. Once they have handed in their cards, read through and answer them with the help of the adult women.

Erasing the Spirit of Fear

This time of change in their bodies is an uncertain time for our daughters. Their bodies are doing something that is totally out of their control. Just like in birth and menopause, we don't know the hour and day it will start, end, etc. It can be a little scary. **There are blank lines in the workbook (SW-p17) for them to write on. Let the girls voice their fears, if they have any.**

NOTE: Here is some optional wisdom to share with the class:

> "For maidenhood, young girls have trepidations about their first cycle coming. They may be anxious because they are not sure what it entails. Maternity is another area where fear grows and expands rapidly. In Menopause, women refuse to understand fully what their body is about to go through, because of the fear that surrounds it as well. Why is this? It is because of the culture we live in, no doubt. In most instances, this is a spirit of fear. It is a fear of the unknown. As humans, we want to control and know everything. That is what makes us comfortable and safe. Well-seasoned Christians will tell you this is not so, that it is not walking in faith, but truly by sight. We need to walk in faith, trusting and knowing that God has ordained these cycles and that they are in His hands! They always have been, and always will be. His grace is sufficient, even for menses, maternity and menopause. Young girls may be scared or fearful because of stories they hear at school or church, or of boys making fun of them, or maybe because they are afraid everyone will know when they are having their menstruation. Pregnant women fear the birth, the pain, and the work of raising children. Menopausal women are scared of the process of their cycle ceasing or waning and their hormones controlling their lives and driving them crazy. We need support, we need our fellow Christian sisters pointing us to God, who alone is wise and merciful."—Doran Richards

We, as humans, like to have control over our bodies. Talk with your class or student about this concept or belief. Some women may take pills to stop their cycle or to manage it, and for true medical needs this is a blessing, but simply for the ability to predict or control your cycle, it might be better to leave some things for the Lord to reveal in His own time. This attitude gives us a spirit of reliance and dependence on One who is larger than life!

Ask and discuss these questions (SW-p17):

- How can we predict the arrival of our period?
- Do we *need* to predict the arrival?
- Is there a balance?
- How can we know what to expect from day to day?

- What does scripture say about dwelling in the past or wanting to know future events?

(SW-p18) Our culture paints a picture of this season of our lives as undesirable and burdensome. Our culture has also taken it to another extreme and worshiped the act of menstruation, the moon, and the body. We need to be aware of what the secular or Western worldview is concerning our cycles so we can be shining examples of Jesus Christ even (or especially) in our cycle, balancing our own perspectives by seeing His design and the need for it.

> **Isaiah 41:10b:** Don't panic. I'm with you. There's no need to fear for I'm your God. I'll give you strength. I'll help you. I'll hold you steady, keep a firm grip on you.

> **2 Timothy 1:7:** God doesn't want us to be shy with his gifts, but bold and loving and sensible.

Mental Health

Young women, as part of maturing, have more pronounced and sensitive feelings concerning their bodies (and what their peers are thinking and doing) and may be dealing with heightened anxiety throughout the process of beginning their cycle and going through bodily changes.

> "Worrying is carrying tomorrow's load with today's strength—carrying two days at once. It is moving into tomorrow ahead of time. Worrying doesn't empty tomorrow of its sorrow, it empties today of its strength." - Corrie ten Boom

> "Anxiety's like a rocking chair. It gives you something to do, but it doesn't get you very far." - Jodi Picoult, *Sing You Home*

> "That's the thing about fear. It can only hang around until faith enters the room, then it's forced to flee." - Mandy Hale

Having fear and anxiety produces chemical and physical reactions in your body. The **fear-tension-pain syndrome** is a known experience during childbirth, but is also a great way to teach them about this phase in their lives as well. There are great resources for alleviating fear and anxiety that includes tapping, or Emotional Freedom Technique (EFT) and also you can release fear through breathing, praying and meditating.

Fear-tension-pain syndrome is a concept formulated by Grantly Dick-Read, MD, (1890-1959) to explain the pain commonly expected and reported in childbirth. The concept proposes that attitudes induce anxiety before labor and cause fear during labor. This is similar to any event in our lives causing anxiety. Our body responds to fear with tension and then eventually turns that constant tension into pain. It is a cycle that we want to recognize and combat with positive affirmations, knowledge, and resources. The more knowledge you have, the better equipped and confident you will be to handle this phase of womanhood.

(SW-p18) Some girls are dealing with pre-existing disorders like anxiety, depression, and trauma from abuse. We have to be keenly aware of the mental stability and well-being of our daughters and we must acknowledge that there could be other factors filtering into what they may be feeling and how they are reacting to growth, maturity, and physical change.

People with these disorders may feel anxious and stressed on a daily basis and for prolonged periods of time. These disorders include:

(SW-p19) **Generalized anxiety disorder** (GAD) is a common anxiety disorder that causes uncontrollable worrying. Sometimes people worry about bad things happening to them or loved ones, and at other times the person may not be able to identify any specific source of worry.

Panic disorder is a condition that manifests as moments of extreme fear, a pounding heart, and shortness of breath, commonly known as panic attacks.

Post-traumatic stress disorder (PTSD) is a condition that causes flashbacks or anxiety as the result of a traumatic experience.

Social phobia is a condition that causes intense feelings of anxiety in situations that involve interacting with others. (It is also known more generally as "social anxiety.")

Obsessive-compulsive disorder (OCD) is a condition that causes repetitive thoughts and the compulsion to complete certain ritual actions in order to feel in control.

It's not always easy, and it often comes down to a choice (graphic in SW-p19):

- Choosing not to allow fear and anxiety to control your life.

- Choosing to guard your heart.

- Choosing to focus your mind on what is truth in the midst of uncertain times.

We might still feel afraid, but we can believe that God is with us. We may not be in control, but we can trust the One who is. We may not know the future, but we can know the God who does.

"So do not fear, for I am with you; do not be dismayed, for I am your God. I will strengthen you and help you; I will uphold you with my righteous right hand." **- Isaiah 41:10**

"When I am afraid, I put my trust in you." **- Psalm 56:3**

"Do not be anxious about anything, but in every situation, by prayer and petition, with thanksgiving, present your requests to God. And the peace of God, which transcends all understanding, will guard your hearts and your minds in Christ Jesus." **- Philippians 4:6-7**

"Peace is what I leave with you; it is my own peace that I give you. I do not give it as the world does. Do not be worried and upset; do not be afraid." **- John 14:27**

"For God has not given us a spirit of fear, but of power and of love and of a sound mind." **- 2 Timothy 1:7**

"There is no fear in love. But perfect love drives out fear, because fear has to do with punishment. The one who fears is not made perfect in love." **- 1 John 4:18**

"When anxiety was great within me, your consolation brought joy to my soul." **- Psalm 94:19**

(SW-p19) "But now, this is what the Lord says...Fear not, for I have redeemed you; I have summoned you by name; you are mine." **- Isaiah 43:1**

"An anxious heart weighs a man down, but a kind word cheers him up." - **Proverbs 12:25**

"Even though I walk through the valley of the shadow of death, I will fear no evil, for you are with me; your rod and your staff, they comfort me." - **Psalm 23:4**

NOTE: Perhaps have each girl (and/or mother) take turns reading the scriptures above aloud.

We will talk more about how to take your thoughts captive. It is one thing to say to a young lady, or anyone, "take your thoughts captive," yet it is another thing to give them actual resources to help them in this activity. Not engaging in negativity is hard work. Scripture is our first resource, knowing that it is alive and feeds our soul. But there are other exercises we can encourage in our daughters (as well as ourselves).

10 Steps to Mastering Your Thoughts and Moods
By Rebecca Chamaa

Like the old saying goes, "Which came first, the chicken or the egg?" That is how it is with our thoughts and our moods. Which came first, the negative thought or the foul mood? No matter which came first, the two go hand in hand. You can become a master at controlling your thoughts and moods by practicing these ten exercises. You can fulfill this passage from Scripture at the same time: We demolish arguments and every pretension that sets itself up against the knowledge of God, and we take captive every thought to make it obedient to Christ. **- 2 Corinthians 10:5 NIV**.

1. Memorize this passage of Scripture and put it into practice:

"…whatever is true, whatever is noble, whatever is right, whatever is pure, whatever is lovely, whatever is admirable—if anything is excellent or praiseworthy—think about such things." **- Philippians 4:8 NIV**

2. Another good way to halt and change the direction of negative thoughts and bad moods is to stop and begin to thank God for all that is good or right in your life. It is hard to be in a bad mood or have negative thoughts when you start to list your blessings. Depending upon the severity of the mood, a short list will probably start to lift your spirits, but if it doesn't, try listing the things we often overlook…dig deep in your heart for what you might have that others long to have (eyesight, hearing, food, clothes, shelter, the ability to walk or bend over, joints that don't ache, etc).

3. Start a hope list. Think about all that you would like to have happen over the next year and write it down. Then think about all the things you would like to have happen over the next six months and write them down. Then make a list of the things you would like to have happen in the next month and write them down. Pick one item from each list and write steps that you can take to make these things a reality. Pray about your hope list and visit it often to make changes, mark progress, and add steps to help you accomplish these things.

4. (SW-p20) Another way to change the course of your thoughts is to stop and ask God to take control of your day. Just give the day over to God and let Him know you need His help. This usually provides some much-needed comfort and the hope that things will begin to change.

5. (SW-p20) Taking action is a great way to lift your spirits. It could be taking action against a dirty house (if you do this one, start with one room, and start with a small chore first so you can see your progress), or it could be starting to work on a project that has been sitting for a long time, or it could be writing a letter. The possibilities for this exercise are endless.

6. Take a walk and use the time to either talk to God, or listen to an audio sermon, Bible on tape, or Christian music. The walk alone should help give your mood a boost, and the time spent worshiping will be an added lift.

7. Write down all the negative thoughts you are having and then spend some time looking through the Bible for verses that oppose your thoughts. A quick and easy way to do this is by buying a book that addresses everyday problems with scriptures. A good one is called *God's Promises for Every Day*, by A.L. Gill, the New Century Version.

8. Say the Lord's Prayer over and over again until you can get through it without having any other thoughts intrude (you might find that you have to say it up to ten times). Start over every time you catch your mind wandering.

9. Think about the people you know and the struggles they are having, or think about people in parts of the world and their struggles. Stop and say a prayer for all those you thought about.

10. Sing your favorite Christian song from beginning to end. Keep singing it until you start to feel better.

If you try all ten exercises, and you find that you still can't shake those negative thoughts or a bad mood, then keep in mind that the real Master is always there to assist you and with His help and guidance and you will be tapped into the ultimate source of joy and strength. You can also call everyone you know and let them know that God created both the chicken and the egg, and the mystery is just His way of "fowling" around!

© *by Rebecca Chamaa. About the Author: Rebecca was a social worker in Washington State for over seven years. Five of those years were spent working with Children and Family Services. She currently lives in Southern California with her husband.*

Taking your thoughts captive is often quoted when we realize the amount of negativity running through our thought process. The evil one, Satan, is oftentimes blamed for our thoughts. In reality, Satan has no authority or space available in our bodies if we are believers and children of God. Only one Spirit inhabits our bodies(God does not share space with Satan!), and that is of the Holy Spirit. Recognizing that our own fleshly thoughts are the culprit to negativity can be eye opening and freeing, knowing we can change our thought processes and switch to more positive thinking and ideals toward ourselves and others.

6 Ways To Take Your Thoughts Captive (from crosswalk.com):

1. **Accept responsibility for your thoughts.** You have the ability to exercise control over your thoughts. God warned Cain to focus his mind on the right things, but Cain chose to think about the wrong things—anger and jealousy—which led to his murderous actions. *Are you*

willing to admit that you can, with God's help, regain control of your thoughts, and think enabling thoughts instead of disabling ones?

2. Your mind—not just your behavior—must change. God calls us to change sinful behavior that does not honor and please Him. Instead of focusing on your outward behavior, work on disciplining your mind, from which the behaviors stem. Allow God to transform you by the renewing of your mind (Rom. 12:2).

3. Think through your problems rather than just react to them. When you experience difficult challenges, you can react to them and think yourself into despair every time. Or you can look forward to the next opportunity and ask yourself what you learned from this failure. Is your first thought *I'll never do anything right?* You don't have to get trapped by disabling thoughts. You are capable of getting out of your shame, despair, hopelessness, and anger by taking control of your thoughts.

4. Take your disabling thoughts captive through confession. Paul urges us to "take captive every thought to make it obedient to Christ" (Rom. 12:21). Confront your disabling thoughts. Turn them over to God and become who He sees you can be. It will take work to take your thoughts captive *each time* they pop into your mind. But it is possible with the help of the Holy Spirit.

5. Choose to focus your thoughts on the right things. We are to think about those things that are "true, noble, right, pure, lovely, and admirable" (Phil. 4:8). When we think on those things, God promises to give us His peace. What a contrast that is to the thoughts of millions of people today. Don't look to a movie, TV show, or how-to formula to accomplish this for you. It takes personal discipline and commitment.

6. It is possible. It is not easy to retrain your thoughts or to respond in new Christ-like ways. Take heart: as God empowers you to focus your mind on the right things, it will become easier. You *can* develop a new frame of reference, based on what is *true, noble, right, pure, lovely, admirable, excellent,* and *praiseworthy.*

Learning how our bodies function and why our bodies change is the first step to erasing anxiety we might have surrounding these changes. Understanding God's design and trusting His good work is essential to finding security and peace about our cycles. Getting the true facts about our cycle is very important!

When we understand why our bodies function the way they do, we are comforted by knowing what to expect next. Having faith in God gives us the knowledge that everything is designed to work together for an ultimate purpose—His purpose. This erases fear and anxiety.

NOTE: In the Student Workbook, there is a place for them to write their favorite way to take thoughts captive.

HORMONES AND MY PERSONAL PROVERBS CHARTING

REVIEW - Go over previous chapters and definitions.

- What is your favorite product to use during your cycle?

- What does the word *mensis* mean or derive from?

- What scripture can you think of that helps you take thoughts captive?

This chapter is about the hormones in your body and conditions that may cause emotional changes to occur during the menstrual cycle. You can review **Diagram 1.5** in **Chapter 1**.

NOTE: Write the definitions from this chapter on the board so they can copy them in **Chapter 4** of their workbook.

Definition of PMS

Premenstrual Syndrome sounds like an illness, doesn't it? Well, it is certainly something we need to be aware of but we do not need to see it as an illness or disease. This "condition" is caused by a higher level of hormonal activity in our bodies before our periods. It may even extend into our actual menstruation time. But it does subside once our cycle starts, and we can ease our PMS by looking at our diet and nutrition and mental well-being.

Just like with any other change in our health condition, there is always a way to treat it with over-the-counter (OTC) medicine. These medicines can be drugs and other types of remedies. Sometimes, in extreme cases, PMS might require these OTC medicines.

Usually we can combat the misconception that menstruation is an illness or disease by focusing on God's perfect design for our bodies. This will enable us to see what our body is doing so that we can work *naturally* to help our bodies cope with the changes taking place within them. Diet, exercise, and nutrition play an important role in the way we feel throughout our cycle and ensures our body will function at its optimal capacity.

Aviva Romm has this information:
> **PMS** is usually due to a combination of factors that lead to hormonal imbalances, imbalances in the stress hormones, and the neurotransmitters (chemicals that control mood).

Underlying factors:

- Nutrient deficiencies (especially B6, vitamin E, vitamin A, calcium, and magnesium)

- Blood sugar dysregulation

- Environmental factors, especially excess estrogen from plastics and other chemical exposures

- Stress (relationship, marital / sexual difficulties; workplace stress, money, etc.)

Thyroid problems can also cause PMS, so have your doctor check your thyroid hormones to make sure these are in proper order. And while you're at it, get your iodine and vitamin D levels checked—when low these can contribute to depression and other related symptoms.

Sometimes, improving one factor alone can improve symptoms, but most often a combination approach of improved diet, improved lifestyle habits (for example, adequate rest, increased exercise, and changed beliefs about menstruation), and herbal and nutritional supplements can help.

These are also areas that you can look into for PMS health:

- **Lifestyle Habits**
- **Herbs**
- **Hormonal Regulators**
- **Stress Relieving Nervines**
- **Adaptogens**
- **Liver Herbs**
- **Chinese Herbs**

The good news about PMS is that once our menstruation actually begins, the symptoms for PMS greatly diminish, if not disappear altogether, due to the hormonal changes that take place naturally. Let's learn about the hormones that can create PMS.

NOTE: Explain what a hormone is—write these definitions on board or have them on a PowerPoint slide so the students can write the vocabulary in their student workbooks:

Hormone: A chemical substance produced in the body's endocrine glands.

Hormones are used at various times in our cycle to do various actions like triggering the next phase. Remember what our phases are? **Review the names of phases with students.**

Women primarily produce two different types of hormones in connection with a menstrual cycle: **Estrogen** and **progesterone**, which are made by the body throughout the reproductive years and are responsible for each monthly period.

Estrogen: Any of several steroid hormones that regulate female reproductive functions. This hormone induces menstruation in women. Estrogen is also important for the maintenance of normal brain function and the development of nerve cells.

Progesterone: A female hormone secreted by the ovaries. It acts to prepare the uterus for pregnancy, to maintain pregnancy, and to promote breast development.

> "The hormone of femininity (estrogen) is more active during the first part of the cycle and reaches its peak just at the time of ovulation. The maternity hormone (progesterone) is more active during the second part of the cycle. Progesterone helps prepare the lining of the uterus to receive a fertilized ovum (egg)." — Ingrid Trobisch in *The Joy of Being a Woman*

If estrogen predominates (or is higher than progesterone) during a cycle, anxiety occurs. If there is more progesterone, depression may be a complaint. There is help available for these issues and we will get to those resources in the coming chapters.

Let's review the phases of our cycle by playing "The Phase Game."

ACTIVITY: The Phase Game (for students and mothers)

Remember the phases from **Chapter 1**? To play this game, you can have the mothers against the daughters or break the daughters up into two groups—or find another creative way to make this interactive and fun for the students.

I am the phase that expels an egg from the ovary. (ovulation)

I am the phase that creates the highest level of hormonal activity. (luteal)

I am the phase that matures the egg sac or follicle. (follicular)

I am the phase that sheds the uterine lining once a month. (menstruation)

I am the phase where you may feel tired and irritable and out-of-sorts emotionally. (luteal)

I am the phase that is about 14 days before your menstruation begins. (ovulation)

I am the phase where the lining of your uterus will begin to thicken and build up. (follicular)

I am the phase that is oftentimes called "Aunt Flo." (menstruation)

I am the phase where you might not see a lot of discharge. (luteal)

I am the stage that requires extra focus on the LORD and His design for me. (luteal)

You can hand out a treat to all players and tell them what a great job they did! (Consider treats that are healthier than candy, like protein bars or granola.)

Charting Your Cycle: My Personal Proverbs (SW-p26)

Introduction for My Personal Proverbs Charting (*first created by Rachel Himelright*):
Welcome to a new and unique way to chart your menstrual cycle! This may be the first method you've tried or a new one for you. Either way, I hope it blesses you as you move through the months of your life and become intimately familiar with the Proverbs and God's miraculous design for your body. This charting system is intended to help you see God in our design and glorify Him as you see your own personal cycle emerge.

The Proverbs in the Bible speak to our human condition, offering guidelines to help us make good decisions in our lives. As women, there is a wealth of information in the Proverbs about what kind of women the Lord seeks to mold us into. I pray as you study them, He will use them to help you trust Him and His miraculous design.

My Personal Proverbs charting system is a valuable tool for many reasons, but the most important one is for you to be knowledgeable about what is happening in your cycle.

Understanding what is happening will drastically decrease the fear and anxiety that might cause your emotions to run wild. Knowledge is power. While charting, you will be pointed to God and His goodness and mercy to us as women. Remember to keep your colored pens and Bible handy!

Instructions for My Personal Proverbs (SW-p27)

You can use regular calendar months in a personal pocket size calendar. Use colored pens to help you see what phase of your cycle you are in. The colors are **red**, **blue**, **green** and **purple**.

We will use four different colored pens for making notations on the calendar pages as our bodies change over the course of our cycle. Colors also represent certain things in the Bible—those definitions have been included here for you to think about. Use your Bible or Bible app as a resource for reading Proverbs that correspond to the various points in your cycle.

Wait for the first day of your period to begin.

When Day One arrives, use a RED marker to write "Prov. 1" on that day on your calendar. Read that Proverb and say a prayer. Invite the LORD into this process and ask Him to be glorified in it. Also note how heavy the flow of your cycle happens to be that day by using the initials "L" for Light, "M" for Medium and "H" for Heavy. This type of charting will help you determine your ability for sports or other activities where this would alter how you feel or your ability to participate.

Continue to mark each day of your monthly cycle using the various colors as indicated below. Read Proverb 2 on Day 2, Proverb 3 on Day 3 and so on. Change the color as your phase changes. Make sure you write down (in the appropriate color) what Proverb you have read that day.

The descriptions for colors indicate physical as well as mental changes taking place. One of those important and most visible changes will be the mucus or discharge coming from your vagina. Don't be afraid of this discharge that God designed. It is there for good reason and it indicates a healthy cycle. It is sometimes non-existent, sometimes light, and yet other times heavier—all indicating your body is changing throughout the whole month. Remember, there is constant renewing taking place!

Your mucous can be checked by noticing what is present on the toilet paper when you wipe after using the bathroom. See the descriptions below that talk about mucus changes.

The colors you will use for the four phases are:

RED – (Blood and Atonement) This is the *Menstruation Phase*. This color will be for the time of bleeding. Begin to use it as soon as you see blood. It can be bright red, dark red, light pink, or brownish in color. Consider doing a devotional on top of the Proverb each day to help you stay focused during this more difficult hormonal period. During this time, you might feel bloated, you might be **cramping** (your uterus is contracting to help expel the lining and blood), and you may be tired. Remember to rest during this phase of your cycle as much as possible.

BLUE (SW-p28)– (Heaven and Heavenly Grace) This is the _Follicular Phase_. This color indicates the time in your cycle prior to ovulation. You may notice a small amount of watery or sticky discharge from your vagina during this phase. Your uterus is building a new lining of blood and one of your ovaries is growing an egg sac. Your estrogen is higher now because your body is working hard to produce an egg. Your spirit should feel joyful and renewed. You have a higher level of energy during this time.

GREEN – (New Life) This is the _Ovulation Phase_. You will use this color to chart when you body is ovulating. The best indicator of ovulation is the amount and consistency of your discharge (also called "cervical mucus"). You will notice the most discharge during this phase; the mucus is slippery, wet, and elastic. It can be clear, white or gold in color. Ovulation (egg release) takes place in this 24-48 hour time frame. Your period will start in about 14-16 days. Your body feels rather good due to your hormones being at high levels (your estrogen is peaking now), though you may also feel some minor cramping or aches as well.

PURPLE – (Richness, Abundance, Infilling of the Holy Spirit) This is the _Luteal Phase_. This phase lasts anywhere from 10 to 14 days and is the time before your period begins. Work with _extra focus_ on the LORD—looking to Him for your strength, joy, and peace—for this is the phase where you might experience PMS or mood swings. Your hormone levels are fluctuating, causing sensitivity or moodiness. You may have a small amount of milky white mucus now. Your breasts may feel sore, heavy, or more tender than usual. This is an important color to chart, marking when you may need MORE grace and love toward those around you!

NOTE: You may not always make it through 31 Proverbs before you are ready to start with the red marker again. The beauty of this exercise is how it allows you to see each of the Proverbs from a different perspective as you go through them at different times in your cycle. Reading one Proverb a day is the key and there is no set place to start.

ACTIVITY: True or False (SW-p29)

Test the students to see what they have learned thus far about their monthly cycle. Do the True or False worksheet together in class or give them a little time to work alone.

Please mark the correct answer:

> When we keep track of our cycle, using a chart, it will help us see how our emotional well-being is doing. **<u>TRUE</u>** or FALSE
>
> During menstruation, the menstrual flow we have consists of all blood. TRUE or **<u>FALSE</u>**
>
> My body is physically affected in only one way during my cycle. TRUE or **<u>FALSE</u>**
>
> My body works better if it is hormonally balanced. **<u>TRUE</u>** or FALSE
>
> PMS stands for Post Menstruation Sickness. TRUE or **<u>FALSE</u>**

Help for Menses & PMS: 7-Day Devotional (SW-p29)

Explain that this devotional is to begin when they are in the **Purple Stage** for charting their cycles and doing their *My Personal Proverbs*. The purple stage, or luteal phase, is up to a week before their period begins. It is when PMS symptoms are most likely to occur. It might even briefly go into the **Red Stage**, when menstruation begins.

The purpose of the **7-Day Devotional** is to keep them focused on the Lord, drawing upon Him in this time of bodily changes that are out of their control. Explain that keeping the Devotional handy during their cycle would be a good idea.

You will see that there are seven days of prayers and scriptures here to help you go through the menstruation phase. Each day of bleeding, meditate on the scriptures for that day, memorize them, and recite them to yourself a few times throughout the day. This will help you through the beginning of your cycle and will establish an important element in your life as a Christian—trusting God's word and applying it to this aspect of being a woman. (**NOTE:** Maybe just read a day or two to give them a taste of what it is and how it is laid out.)

DAY 1

Prayer: Lord, I come before You today, the first day of my bleeding, to ask You to strengthen my heart, body, and soul. I pray that the Holy Spirit guides me through the next few days as I experience this awesome design of Yours to cleanse my body. I am grateful, God, for this process and praise Your holy name! I pray for continued support during this time, in Jesus' name I pray, Amen.

Scriptures:

The name of the Lord is a strong tower; the righteous run to it and are safe. God's name is a place of protection—good people can run there and be safe. **- Proverbs 18:10**

The wise counsel God gives when I'm awake is confirmed by my sleeping heart. Day and night I'll stick with God; I've got a good thing going and I'm not letting go. **- Psalm 16:7-8**

DAY 2

Prayer: Oh, Holy Spirit, help me in my distress and discomfort. Help me, O' God, see the beauty of Your beautiful design for me as a woman. I thank You this day that You have given me the gift of menstruation so that my body can cleanse itself and lend my body to health. I pray Your Spirit to teach me how to be content and patient with this process. Help me to be Christ-like in all I do and say this day, when it is extra hard to be kind due to my hormones fluctuating so! I pray all of this in Jesus' name, Amen.

Scriptures:

I'm sure now I'll see God's goodness in the exuberant earth. Stay with God! Take heart. Don't quit. I'll say it again: Stay with God. **- Psalm 27:14**

God gives a hand to those down on their luck, gives a fresh start to those ready to quit. **- Psalm 145:14**

DAY 3 (SW-p30)

Prayer: This is the third day of my menstruation and I seek Your holy face to help me in the most difficult part of the bleeding process. Lord, give me thoughts of peace and joy with contentment this day. Help me in spite of my discomfort to be Christ-like in all I do and say, helping me give glory to God, even now. I pray, Lord, for Your help in seeing my sinful nature. Help me to repent and go and sin no more. Thank You God for loving me still, like only a loving Father could. I pray this in Jesus' name, Amen.

Scriptures:

I pray to God—my life a prayer— and wait for what he'll say and do. My life's on the line before God, my Lord, waiting and watching till morning, waiting and watching till morning. **- Psalm 130:5-6**

So be content with who you are, and don't put on airs. God's strong hand is on you; he'll promote you at the right time. Live carefree before God; he is most careful with you. **- I Peter 5:7**

DAY 4

Prayer: I ask you, Lord, to wrap Your arms around me and let me feel Your holy presence. I love the design You have made in my body to work the way it does. I will be content in knowing all things are for a purpose and for Your good reason. Be with me as I do my duties today, giving me a spirit of sound mind, body, and soul so that I can let my light so shine before others, giving You all the glory, honor, and praise! I pray this in Jesus' name, Amen.

Scriptures:

"This is God's Message, the God who made earth, made it livable and lasting, known everywhere as *God*: 'Call to me and I will answer you. I'll tell you marvelous and wondrous things that you could never figure out on your own.'" **- Jeremiah 33:3**

So let God work his will in you. Yell a loud *no* to the Devil and watch him scamper. Say a quiet *yes* to God and he'll be there in no time. Quit dabbling in sin. Purify your inner life. Quit playing the field. Hit bottom, and cry your eyes out. The fun and games are over. Get serious, really serious. Get down on your knees before the Master; it's the only way you'll get on your feet. **- James 4:7-10**

DAY 5

Prayer: Dear Lord, I love You and seek Your face forever more. I praise you, Lord, for Your loving kindness toward me. Help me, Holy Spirit to see and feel You this day, renewing a steadfast spirit in me and washing me whiter than snow. Jesus, I thank You for Your example of walking in love toward one another. Help me do that this day when my hormones are working hard inside my body. I am thankful for the work You are doing within me, grateful that You have a design for us as women and it is good. I pray this in Jesus' name, Amen.

Scriptures:

I call to God; God will help me. At dusk, dawn, and noon I sigh deep sighs—he hears, he rescues. My life is well and whole, secure in the middle of danger even while thousands are lined up against me. God hears it all, and from his judge's bench puts them in their place. But, set in their ways, they won't change; they pay him no mind. **- Psalm 55:16-19**

A cheerful disposition is good for your health; gloom and doom leave you bone-tired. **- Proverbs 17:22**

DAY 6

Prayer: Lord, it is nearing the end of my bleeding for this month and I am always amazed at the beauty of Your design to have my body perform this cleansing. I pray for Your guidance as I finish this cycle; bringing me through with a happy heart and as a good example of Christ, even in a time when it is harder to do so. I acknowledge You in all I do and pray the Holy Spirit teaches me how I can be better at doing Your will each and every day. Thank You, dear God, for loving me and protecting me each day. I pray this in Jesus' name, Amen.

Scriptures:

A devout life does bring wealth, but it's the rich simplicity of being yourself before God. Since we entered the world penniless and will leave it penniless, if we have bread on the table and shoes on our feet, that's enough. **- I Timothy 6:6-8**

"You're blessed when you're content with just who you are—no more, no less. That's the moment you find yourselves proud owners of everything that can't be bought." **- Matthew 5:5**

DAY 7

Prayer: Ah, Lord God—what a beautiful day you have given me. This is the day the Lord has made and I will be happy and rejoice in it! Thank You for Your mercy that endures forever and strength that surpasses all understanding. I praise You for Your love that has brought me through this week of my life. I pray for You to carry me through until my next cycle begins. Help me, Lord, to follow You every day of my life, doing Your will, not mine—by the power of the Holy Spirit working within me. Great is thy faithfulness! I pray this in Jesus' name, Amen!

Scriptures:

The aspirations of good people end in celebration; the ambitions of bad people crash. **- Proverbs 10:28**

So let's not allow ourselves to get fatigued doing good. At the right time we will harvest a good crop if we don't give up, or quit. Right now, therefore, every time we get the chance, let us work for the benefit of all, starting with the people closest to us in the community of faith. **- Galatians 6:9-10**

Chapter 5
PHYSICAL CHANGES & WHOLE–BODY WELLNESS

REVIEW (SW-p33)

Go over previous chapters if you feel it is needed before introducing new information about changes in the mind, body, and soul.

- What hormones are working in your body all month long?
- What is the importance of charting your cycle?

This week's discussion is about other ways hormones help to change our bodies during our cycles. We will talk about the body and how it begins to change (such as how it affects our skin).

NOTE: Menarche, which is the first occurrence of menstruation, can begin as early as 2 years before your actual menstrual flow.

Physical Changes

When talking about bodily changes for beginning menstruation and puberty, you can have a little scripture study or discussion about changes. First start with how God never changes. He is constant, and His design is good. We are the ones that change, and that is a good thing!

> "Appreciate your pastoral leaders who gave you the Word of God. Take a good look at the way they live, and let their faithfulness instruct you, as well as their truthfulness. There should be a consistency that runs through us all. For Jesus doesn't change— yesterday, today, tomorrow, he's always totally himself." ~ Hebrews 13:8, The Message

> "We can embrace change by knowing we serve an unchanging God." ~ David Jeremiah

> "God's unchanging word equips us to understand His ways and to stand firm in faith." ~ Euginia Herlihy

> "God is like a mirror, consistent, stable, unchanging; reflecting His image of us, that is always changing." ~ Anthony Liccione

> "So we do not lose heart. Though our outer self is wasting away, our inner self is being renewed day by day. For this light momentary affliction is preparing for us an eternal weight of glory beyond all comparison, as we look not to the things that are seen but to the things that are unseen. For the things that are seen are transient, but the things that are unseen are eternal." 2 Corinthians 4:16-18 ESV

Thoughts about change, and changing:

- Each day we are changing, being sanctified, and renewed.

- Only Jesus doesn't change.

- Change is a part of who we are, who we were created to be, who we will become.

- Physical changes are signs of internal changes.

- Physical changes, internal and external, are for our good.

- Change is usually for the better.

- Change can be hard and confusing.

Discussion Questions:

- How would you encourage young girls about changes happening to their bodies?

- How would you enlighten them that they can embrace them, instead of being

confused or anxious about them?

- How do you personally handle change?

First, we will talk about some physical changes that occur before our menstruation begins for the first time. Growing up means experiencing changes in the process of becoming mature. Let's discuss some of those changes now.

Before your menses occurs, your body will undergo some physical changes. Most common are breast changes, growing of body hair, having a growth spurt, and (probably) skin changes. These are all normal and to be expected, not to be feared. Every woman you know went through these changes too.

Ask the class, "What other changes can you come up with that we haven't talked about yet?" Perhaps oily hair, hips are expanding a little more, and any others additions volunteered by the class.

Breast Development
The first physical sign of puberty in girls is usually breast development. This often begins as a firm, tender lump under the center of the areola of one or both breasts, occurring, on average, at about age 10. Within 6-12 months, the swelling has clearly begun in both sides. The lump has softened, and can be seen extending beyond the edges of the areolae. In another 12 months, the breasts are approaching mature size and shape.

Breast development can be a tender and sometimes painful growth stage. Be aware that it is normal for some girls to experience discomfort. One side of your body will look different than the other. The breasts are not identical twins; they are unique and may have differences, both subtle and more marked. For example, the nipples could protrude one upward and one downward. Another example would be to have what are called "inverted nipples" or flat nipples. (Inverted nipples are something to be aware of, but don't usually cause any problems. This is simply information that may serve you when going through childbearing and through nursing.) God has created each of us very uniquely and our differences are what make us individuals. We can be content that His design for us is good.

When the breasts begin to form, it is a good idea to purchase a few bras. Some reasons for that are:

- The breasts are mainly made of fat; there is not much muscle to support them. A well-fitted bra will support the breasts so that there is no discomfort at the end of the day.

- When we get cold or chilled, our nipples can stick out and become prominent. A bra will help hide this from others, keeping modesty intact.

- Our breasts were made to feed babies someday. They are also meant to be kept private. A bra will help us to feel covered up.

Purchasing and buying a bra can be daunting with all the choices available now. There are companies that size correctly and have more age appropriate options. Some also believe that wearing a bra is not important or necessary.

NOTE: Let students know that they should discuss underwire bras with their mothers—they have the potential to cause long-term harm if worn daily. You have lymph nodes under your arms on the sides of your breasts that should be unconstricted.

Pubic Hair (SW-p34)
Pubic hair is often the second change in puberty. These hairs grow between the legs and are usually visible first along the labia. The hair will eventually cover the labia and the surrounding area (the "bikini area").

Pubic hair will start off being soft and very fine, gradually becoming more coarse and thick. You will also notice some hair growing under your arms. The hair on your legs gets thicker too. All of these changes are normal and to be expected. Most of our whole body is protected with fine hairs. For example: our arms, inside our nose, our fingers, etc.

Point out to the students that hair is used to protect us and to filter out bad elements or germs. Just like our eyelashes, hair on our head and even the hair on a cob of corn! God is so good to give us protection!

In only about 15% of girls, the pubic hair appears <u>before</u> breast development begins, so don't worry if you see hair without beginning breast development. You will get both hair and breasts.

Body Odor
You will experience many changes in your body and increased or changed body odor may be one of them. There are rising hormones levels that can change the fatty acid composition of perspiration (your sweat), resulting in a more "adult" smell. This is an ideal time to start wearing deodorant. Your mother will help you decide when you can start using it.

NOTE: Point out that **antiperspirant** is meant to lessen or stop perspiration and **deodorant** is used to cover or neutralize odor. I don't personally recommend antiperspirants because our bodies were meant to sweat and release toxins through our skin, something antiperspirants can interfere with.

To combat odor (SW-p35):

- Bathing daily is suggested.

- Wear a deodorant with as many natural ingredients as possible.

- Wear clean underwear and change them often.

Your skin has two types of sweat glands: eccrine and apocrine. Eccrine glands occur over most of your body and open directly onto the surface of your skin. Apocrine glands open into the hair follicle, leading to the surface of the skin. Apocrine glands develop in areas abundant in hair follicles, such as on your scalp, armpits and groin. - Mayo Clinic

The area "down there" is dark, moist, and warm, which can be an ideal climate for yeast infections and uncleanliness to thrive and cause havoc. Getting used to these new habits may take some time and adjustment. Keeping yourself clean is a job that takes maturity and you will get to this level of newfound maturity through a process; it doesn't happen overnight. Be patient with your body and try to work with it by using prayer and asking guidance from the Holy Spirit. He will not leave you nor forsake you during this time.

NOTE: In their Student Workbook they have a space to write why they believe their body odor could be stronger because of hormonal activity.

Skin Changes
Another hormonal change is increased secretion of oil from the skin. This means a higher chance that acne will occur. Acne is the term for clogged pores (blackheads and whiteheads) that become inflamed and appear raised and red, also knowns as pimples. You can get pimples on the face, neck, chest, back, shoulders and even the upper arms. Acne affects most teenagers to some extent and can even continue into adulthood. The need for staying clean and washing yourself more frequently will help you avoid acne during this time.

Sandi Queen in *From Girl…To Woman* states:

> "Your skin will change—it will probably become oilier, and you may get some pimples. Praise the LORD! This is evidence that your hormones are working, as God intended!"

Be careful when washing and cleansing your face daily; too much cleansing can lead to more issues and acne. You want to try different mild cleansers until you find the one that works best for you, keeping in mind that the tissue on your face is sensitive. Some find using coconut oil as a moisturizer helpful, however some find it more drying to the face or pore clogging if you already have very oily skin. We all have different oil and pH levels on our face, so it might take some trial and error to find out what works for your face cleansing. You may need different types of cleanser at different times of the month—as your body changes throughout the month, so does your oil or dryness levels.

Peer Influence (SW-p36)
Throughout puberty, our daughters are not only going through bodily / physical changes, but through emotional stages as well. Their peers begin to have much more influence in their daily lives and their social circles are likely discussing areas of health and well-being. Be prepared to have discussions

and conversations with your daughter ahead of time and be clear about what is appropriate and what is not an appropriate conversation to have with peers. Setting boundaries early will also encourage your child to have open communication with you throughout their teen years. There are a lot of taboos and misinformation out there concerning bodily changes and options for best health and maturation.

> *"Peer influence is a dominant psychosocial issue during adolescence, especially during the early stages. Young teens are highly cognizant of their physical appearance and social behaviors, seeking acceptance within a peer group."* – "Chapter 1: Adolescent Growth and Development" in *Guidelines for Adolescent Nutrition Services* by Jamie Stang, PhD, and Mary Story, PhD.

A note to the mothers/guardians: Other women and girls will have different experiences and knowledge from different sources which they might share with your daughter. Or they may not have information at all about cycles and menstruation and want your daughter to share her information with them. Discuss with your daughter how everyone will be at different levels of understanding, and if anything is ever confusing to come to you for answers. Boys can also be ignorant about puberty in girls and most will not understand the process correctly unless they have been educated by a parent.

Body Image

As your daughter matures and her body changes, she is going to be highly aware of the changes taking place. Maybe not all the changes at once, but she will be aware that she is growing taller, her hips may be widening, her hair getting oilier, etc. This is an age where they are very self-conscious.

> *"Average weight gains during puberty among females are between 15-55 lb (7-25 kg), with a mean gain of 38.5 lb (17.5 kg). Weight gain slows around the time of menarche, but will continue into late adolescence. Adolescent females may gain as much as 14 lb (6.3 kg) during the latter half of adolescence." –Adolescent Growth and Development* by Jamie Stang and Mary Story

The best example of acceptance and healthy body image comes from you. Mothers have influence like no other in this area, so exercise that influence for the wellbeing of your child by presenting your own body image as positive, individual, and unique.

NOTE: In the Student Workbook (SW-p36) there are blank lines for the girls to write write out how they can be "Positive about body image" and "Does comparison to others help us".

Body Alignment

Your body's alignment can affect your overall health as a woman. How we carry ourselves has impact on our pelvic floor and female reproductive organs. If we are always in a forward position, where our weight is mostly carried on the upper part of our feet (the balls of the feet), then we are out of natural alignment. The weight of your body, when standing, should be equally spread across your feet, with the back (heel) of the feet carrying most of the stress. That way, the pelvis is aligned and tilted the correct way. Be mindful of this and practice standing with your weight properly distributed, with feet firmly planted, which will help you stay aware of where the weight is shifted.

"Alignment isn't something that sounds fun. Therefore, most people, especially teen girls, are not thinking about how they hold their body day in and day out and it is affecting their overall health. The way our body is aligned (or not aligned) affects every cell, every system, every bone, and every muscle of our body. When we are in good alignment, it creates a foundation for better health in the future. Alignment gives our bodies a winning chance at combating the negative effects that aging and stress have on the body. It allows us to move well, sleep well, and live well." — Christina Mroz, Holy Yoga (www.holyyoga.net)

ACTIVITY: Check Alignment

Have the students stand up with hands relaxed at their sides. Talk about how the weight of their bodies should be over the heel of the foot. The pelvic bone (have them feel that on their own body) and their hip bone should both be vertical, not tipping forward or backward. Once they have correct posture, have them put weight on their toes or the front of their feet to feel the difference. Show them with your body the correct alignment. Go here to watch video for instructions on how to do that: https://youtu.be/fXkXW3zW3Y4

Chapter 6
STORY SHARING

REVIEW (SW-p39) - Go over previous chapters and definitions if you feel it is helpful.

- Why is alignment important?
- How long will it take your body to develop breasts and pubic hair?

Story sharing is important and makes this topic easier to discuss comfortably, instead of showing it as a medical event or something frightening. **(Note: There is a coloring page in the student workbooks of a woman touching the hem of Jesus—have them color this while sharing stories.)**

ACTIVITY: Share Your Story

To begin this story sharing time, tell the story of how your menstruation began. What was your experience like? This will help break the ice and encourage other mothers to share their stories. Then read the story below and discuss it as a group. Encourage the girls to ask questions or give comments with each story.

Jesus and the Woman with Bleeding

This is a beautiful story of a woman's faith in our LORD. She looked to Jesus in her time of bleeding to heal her and be her strength. We ought to look at this as an example, meditate on it, and see how we can benefit from looking to Jesus for our regular monthly cycle and menstruation time. This story comes from **Mark 5:25-34:**

> A woman who had suffered a condition of hemorrhaging for twelve years—a long succession of physicians had treated her, and treated her badly, taking all her money and leaving her worse off than before—had heard about Jesus. She slipped in from behind and touched his robe. She was thinking to herself, "If I can put a finger on his robe, I can get well." The moment she did it, the flow of blood dried up. She could feel the change and knew her plague was over and done with.
>
> At the same moment, Jesus felt energy discharging from him. He turned around to the crowd and asked, "Who touched my robe?" His disciples said, "What are you talking about? With this crowd pushing and jostling you, you're asking, 'Who touched me?' Dozens have touched you!" But he went on asking, looking around to see who had done it. The woman, knowing what had happened, knowing she was the one, stepped up in fear and trembling, knelt before him, and gave him the whole story. Jesus said to her, "Daughter, you took a risk of faith, and now you're healed and whole. Live well, live blessed! Be healed of your plague."

We learn from other women's stories that every girl will have a different experience. Girls will start their menstruation at various ages and under different circumstances. What we learn from our mothers and those around us truly affects how we view menstruation and how we adjust to the change in our lives.

History of Menses (SW-p40)

Let's talk about the history of menses. It is interesting to look at other cultures and the history surrounding menstruation. Let us remember we are Christians and we are to see our cycle in God's light and seek to glorify Him in this design for us.

Although most of the ancient cultures recognized the cyclic nature of menses and its relationship to the moon cycles, there was widespread lack of knowledge of our bodily functions in general. This lack of knowledge, or ignorance, led to seeing it as a mystery, a secret—and it became a part of spiritual rituals. Most cultures feared it. A few tribes of people believed it had creative, life-giving powers and saw it as a good thing. Their lack of knowledge led to assuming and creating definitions that may or may not have been true.

The Christian church contributed to the negative attitude of menses, framing it as:

- a secret;
- a dirty sickness that must to be endured and hidden;
- an embarrassment or a curse;
- shame and humiliation;
- punishment for sin, bad thoughts, and guilt.

Unfortunately, this negative attitude toward God's design for women is still present today. We can begin to make a positive change in the way we view menstruation as we learn about menses and see it through the lens of God's perfect plan for us. We can make a difference in our community by always seeking God and being Christ-like examples, even in our cycle.

Here are some facts about menstruation and the calendar:

- Chinese women established a lunar calendar 3,000 years ago.
- Mayan women understood the famous Mayan calendar was based on menstrual cycles.
- Romans called a woman's time of bleeding "menstruation," meaning *knowledge of the menses*.
- In Gaelic, "menstruation" and "calendar" are the same word.

Different Cultures (SW-p41)

Social scientist Aru Bhatiya offers this perspective on menstruation in various cultures:

> "All religions of the world have placed restrictions on menstruating women. Be it Judaism,

> Christianity, Islam, Hinduism, or Buddhism. Sikhism is the only religion where the scriptures condemn sexism and don't impose any restriction on menstruating women."

> "We can see that similar taboos exist across religions and cultures. Some of the most consistent practices followed include isolation, exclusion from religious activities. Women are still prohibited even by the 'modern' religions to enter the temples. Also what is common in all religion is the age-old idea of spiritual impurity, which doesn't seem to go. In society, one tries to avoid the subject of menstruation.

We want to teach our daughters that menstruation looks vastly different in different cultures. The United States has resources, tools, gear, and accessibility that many other cultures and countries may not have.

Other cultures saw the moon's connection in women's cycles:

- Native Americans prayed to the moon for help with an irregular cycle.

- Bahloo, an Aboriginal moon deity, was thought to help create girl babies.

- Maori of New Zealand called menstruation "mata marama" (or "moon sickness").

- Some Indian cultures used the same word for moon and menstrual blood.

Remember, the word menstruation comes from the Latin and Greek words for "month" and "moon." Just like we are not to worship the sun because it warms us, tans us, and provides us light, we are also not to worship the moon for its connection to our cycles.

> "The menstrual process in itself, regardless of its ramifications, must be strange indeed when the physiological bases are unknown. It appears to be a bleeding recurring every twenty-eight days, in the absence of any visible wound or apparent injury to explain it. It occurs exclusively in females, disappearing during pregnancy, and terminating during middle age. Various theories are presented by primitive peoples to explain the cause of menstruation. A common theme is the moon as precipitator of the flow, for lunar cyclical phases have recognized parallel in the menstrual cycle."—Rita E. Montgomery, "A Cross-Cultural Study of Menstruation, Menstrual Taboos, and Related Social Variables."

(SW-p40) These descriptions of different cultures are to give you a picture that women and girls have been cycling since time began, all over the world, and that their God-given functions were not always accepted or welcomed. Here are some cultural approaches to menstruation as shared by Jane Bennet in her book *A Blessing Not a Curse*:

- If a Persian woman's cycle lasted more than 4 days, she was whipped 100 lashes and sent into isolation; if longer, she got 400 lashes. They believed she was possessed by a bad spirit and purification by whip-lashing was thought to be the cure!

- In Andaman Island culture, at menarche (the beginning of menstruation), the parents wept for their daughter's shame.

- In Bathe, a menstruating woman was placed in isolation for three days in a special hut. She was forced to sit very still and was not allowed to sleep, lie down, or speak.

- Some Indian villages prized blood as a powerful substance.

- The Hindu woman was untouchable in menses. One was not permitted to touch her or look at her.

- In China, poetic words were used to describe menstruation: red flood, red snow, peach-flower flow. During menses, women were separated, and they performed no cooking, family duties, or religious rites.

- A Muslim woman recited an article of faith in ritual; there was no fasting, no daily prayers or touching of the Koran. She was subordinate to men because of her menstruation.

Our goal is to get back to God's design for us, regardless of the country we live in, or time period we grow up in, and acknowledge how we are fearfully and wonderfully made. God has created us to endure and to understand the process of our cycle for our health!

> "God equipped women with the capacity to carry life and to give birth. But the gift of menstruation extends for years before and after childbirth, and to women who may not ever have children. This cycle serves us beyond reproduction. Menstruation offers us our body's own calendar, a physical reminder of the need to push ourselves and work and also to rest and reflect."—Amy F. Davis Abdallah, "How I Learned to Love My Period."

ACTIVITY: Word Scramble Game (SW-p43)

Time to play a game! This game will help us review what we have learned so far. It will enable us to really learn the terminology surrounding this season in our lives. It will also be a little break from our listening.

Here is a list of words to unscramble. Have the class split up in two teams or the girls can play this game individually to see who can get the most in a certain amount of time. Or, have the mothers play against the daughters! If you are doing this individually with your daughter, simply let her work on these for about 5 minutes to see if she can figure them out.

16 Word Answers

PAFLAILON EBTUS [fallopian tubes]

VCREXI [cervix]

YVROA [ovary]

RESUTU [uterus]

SOHENOMR [hormones]

TEREGSON [estrogen]

ODBLO [blood]

TNOIVOLUA [ovulation]

GEG CSA [egg sac]

NOITTRUASNEM [menstruation]

SBSAERT [breasts]

CUPBI IRAH [pubic hair]

SMESEN [menses]

HLCOT ADPS [cloth pads]

ROLUALIFC [follicular]

MPTNRUERLAES [premenstrual]

Close out this chapter by asking if there are any questions or comments about the information presented thus far. Engage in conversations with the thoughts or comments shared.

Chapter 7
HEALTH & REJUVENATION

REVIEW (SW-p44)

- What did you learn about the history of menstruation and different cultures?

- Are you thankful for the resources you have today?

DISCLAIMER: The following information is for educational purposes only and the companies and individuals providing this information are not engaged in rendering medical advice or treatment. If you feel that you have a health problem, you should seek the advice of a medical professional.

Diet, Nutrition & Exercise

Lead a discussion about how diet and nutrition play key roles in the overall well-being of our bodies and cycle health. The foods we eat, what we drink daily, what supplements we consume and our activity levels all affect everything about us, including our cycles. It is important to know what foods bring us energy and which ones diminish energy. Eating certain foods at the right time in our cycle can really help improve our mood, vigor, and overall feeling of well-being.

Iron Levels

Iron levels in our body are a special nutritional concern. There is a particular need to maintain healthy iron levels during a woman's years of menstruation. On average, women lose about ¼ cup of blood at each menstrual cycle and women with a heavier flow may lose even more. Since iron travels through the blood, some of iron is lost with the shedding of blood.

Iron is essential for hemoglobin formation (blood volume) and for the effective circulation of oxygen throughout the body. Without adequate levels of iron in the blood, you will be left feeling lethargic and tired, particularly around your time of bleeding.

The best way to obtain nutrients is through food, since it enables us to get the maximum benefit from those nutrients. However, our soils are depleted and not as nutrient dense as they have been in the past, so sometimes other means are necessary to absorb the vitamins and minerals our bodies need.

Good sources of iron include:

- Spinach

- Beans (soybeans, white beans, lentils, kidney beans, chickpeas)

- Clams and oysters

- Apricots, dried

- Prunes, raisins

- Wheat germ

- Meats (beef, duck, lamb)

- Organ meats (liver, giblets)

- Nettles tea or tincture

- Kale, dandelion, and yellow dock

NOTE: It helps to eat foods rich in vitamin C—like oranges and tomatoes—at the same time as an iron-rich food. Vitamin C helps your body absorb iron more efficiently.

> "Foods of high acidity, including yogurt and those rich in vitamin C, increase the body's ability to absorb iron." —Nikki Goldbeck, *As You Eat So Your Baby Grows*

If your diet is not rich in these foods listed, consider taking an iron supplement. Floridix (available from the health food store) is a time-tested, non-constipating, and well-known liquid iron and vitamin supplement. It helps prevent iron deficiency and will greatly increase your energy, health, and well-being. There are other brands in the marketplace that are similar. A supplement that is liver based, such as Enzymatic Therapy Energizing Iron™ with Eleuthero Description, is available on Amazon.com.

Your Diet & Nutrition (SW-p45)
by Aviva Romm, MD, Midwife, Herbalist (From https://avivaromm.com/pms/)

> "Healthy eating is one of the best things you can do for yourself. To ensure that your diet provides all of the nutrients you need, eat a variety of foods and balance the food you eat with exercise.

> Here's where a plant-based diet can make a huge difference, so go Mediterranean-style if PMS is getting to you. A daily dose of dark leafy greens such as kale, collards, and broccoli, as well as good quality fats, are your ticket to the happier hormone party! The high fiber content of vegetables can help the body to effectively eliminate excessive hormones from the intestine, particularly estrogen, while adequate intake of legumes can support the production of hormones when there is a deficiency. Keep dairy products to a minimum to avoid any excess hormones coming into your system. Include cold-water fish (such as salmon and other low-mercury fish) a couple of times a week or take a high-quality fish oil supplement. Dietary fats should come from olive oil, avocados, coconut oil, hemp oil, and other high-quality oils.

> Women with PMS consume significantly more sugar, dairy products, salt, and refined carbohydrates than those who do not experience it. Caffeine intake has also been linked to premenstrual discomforts, especially breast tenderness. Cutting out sugar, all white-flour products, and caffeinated items such as coffee, black tea, and sodas may be hard to do but can go a long way to relieve symptoms. Interestingly, dark chocolate (62% cacao or greater) is the exception to the caffeine rule—it can help improve mood and prevent or relieve depression.

> Adequate protein and fat at each meal will keep your blood sugar at a nice neutral hum—

exactly where you want it to be to avoid the ups and downs of PMS and the roller coaster ride of imbalanced blood sugar—a gnarly combination!

In addition to a healthy diet, several supplements are beneficial in reducing PMS, particularly for improvement of mood, reduction of bloating, and reduction of breast tenderness. These include:

- Calcium citrate (up to 1,200 mg per day)

- Magnesium citrate or glycinate (400 mg per day)

- Vitamin B6 (50 mg per day as part of a B-complex supplement)

- Vitamin E (400 IU per day)

- (SW-p44) DIM (Diindolylmethane) standardized to 25 mg of 25% diindolylmethane, from *Brassicacae* vegetables

- Sulforophane (from Broccoli sprout concentrate) 800 mcg

- Flax seed, 2 TBS fresh ground daily

Evening primrose oil is commonly recommended by herbalists, in a dosage range of 1,500 to 3,000 mg daily, as part of a treatment protocol for PMS. Unfortunately, most clinical trials have failed to show consistent benefit. Nonetheless, increased fatty acid intake has been associated with improved mood when there is depression, and evening primrose is not harmful, making it a practical addition to a treatment plan until further research proves or disproves its benefits.

Drinking a lot of water is a key element in maintaining your health. Water is replenishing and nourishing. Drink at least 8 glasses per day."

Here is some additional direction that can help you choose your meals and snacks each day:

What Does 'Eat a Good Diet' Mean?

By Vickie Frances

"Avoid sugar and all sweeteners, white flour, and white rice. Over and over these items have been shown to cause many health problems. When you do eat them, try to limit yourself to just a bite or two. Non-instant whole grains and brown rice have approximately 300 times the nutrition than the white varieties.

You should choose "nutrient dense" foods for your growing body. At every meal you should have a protein source the size of your palm and at least two vegetables. Protein comes from meat, eggs & dairy.

Avoid soy products as they have something called "estrogen-like compounds," which are not good for your changing hormones. It is important to learn to eat many different kinds of vegetables. Also avoid fried or overcooked vegetables. It is important to eat dark green leafy vegetables at least two times in a week. Those are things like collards, kale, mustard greens, and the most popular: spinach and romaine lettuce. You should try to limit starchy vegetables such as white potatoes and yams to three times a week.

There is a lot of discussion these days about "low fat". As a growing and developing young woman, you should not eat a low-fat diet. It is important, though, to avoid certain fats and concentrate on others. You should avoid margarine, soy oil, vegetable oil, and oils that are not "cold pressed". Some good oils to focus on are olive oil, sunflower oil, safflower oil, and butter. The fats in dairy products and nuts are good for you, too. A lot of people really concerned about good health are adding a spoonful of cod liver oil to their diet every evening. It does taste yucky (unless you like the taste of fish), but the benefits are so important, most of us don't care. Some oils become very bad for you if they are heated to high temperatures, such as for frying.

(SW-p47) You should try to have what is called a varied diet, which means it is one where you eat lots of different kinds of good-for-you foods over the course of a week, so you are providing your body with many different kinds of nutrients. By eating lots of different things, you won't get bored. And don't forget about nuts and seeds. You should limit dried fruit, however, because they contain concentrated sugars. Rather, eat your fruit fresh and whole; a piece or two or a cup of berries a day is a good option—they make great snacks.

Another idea is adding nuts, dried berries, cheese, meat, or eggs to salads. Or try fun things like adding dried cranberries to carrots you are cooking. You can put snacks that are good for you in small containers or ziplock bags, so you won't be tempted by the wrong foods when you are out.

Also remember that water is very important! Avoid drinks that have a lot of sugar like sodas and even sports drinks. Fruit juices sound like a good idea, but they have too much sugar too.

Have fun experimenting with all the yummy things God provided for us to eat!"

Herbs for Your Cycle Health

We will go over a few herbs that will be helpful during your whole monthly cycle and for your health overall. As with medical remedies, herbal remedies should be researched and studied before using. These suggestions are not medical prescriptions and should be used as suggestions.

The four herbs we will explore in depth are:

Nettles

Oat Straw

Red Raspberry Leaf

Alfalfa

ACTIVITY: Sample Herbs to Pass Around

Have sample bags of each herb that you can pass around and let the students and their mothers smell and feel. It will help them remember the information and details for each herb and its properties. This will be the first time some of your attendees will be introduced to herbs. Keep this in mind when teaching. When introducing one herb, pass that bag around while speaking about that particular one.

NORA Tea

Preparation of NORA Tea
(This recipe is also found in the section **Setting Up the Workshop** at the beginning of this Teacher's Guide.)

Herbs are best absorbed into the body and blood stream via liquid. Tea is a great way to get the highest nutritional value from the herbs. We suggest drinking NORA tea. Below you will find information about the herbs in the tea and why they are beneficial to you.

NORA tea is an important part of your women's health. It stimulates your system to optimal health, optimizes mineral absorption, guards against anemia, and maximizes the health of the liver, thereby helping to prevent or minimize many common complaints.

NORA tea consists of four ingredients: **Nettles, Oat Straw, Raspberry Leaf, & Alfalfa.** You can drink this tea daily, up to a quart a day. Drinking throughout the month will enable you to stay toned and strong. If you cannot drink daily, consider drinking the tea a week before your cycle is known to begin.

Preparation of NORA Tea (SW-p48):

- (In the evening) Place a half an inch the of herbs in the bottom of a quart size canning jar (a handful or two). Experiment with the amount of herb and strength of the taste to find what works for you. But please make sure there is at least approximately 1/2 an inch in the jar.

- Fill the jar to 1/2 to 3/4 of an inch from the top with boiling water. Stir the herbs down into the water so that they are all wet and mixed in and not floating.

- Cover the jar with a lid or small plate to retain the essential oils and let sit overnight. In the morning, strain using a small mesh strainer into another canning jar or preferred container and your "tea" (technically an infusion, a concentrated tea) is now ready.

- Feel free to experiment so that you are sure to drink it frequently. To sweeten, add honey or other natural sweeteners like coconut sugar, stevia, etc. You can add ice, or fresh lemons, or lemonade.

Herbs in NORA Tea

Nettles:

Urtica Dioica

Active Ingredients: Histamine, Tannin, Saponins, Acetylcholine Formic Acid, Sterols, Chlorophyll, Glucoquinine, Serotonin, Iron, & Vitamin A, C, D, and K in an easily absorbable form, very high in minerals, including silicon.

Actions: Astringent, diuretic, nutritive, detoxifier, galactagogue, decongestant, hypoglycemic & tonic. ("Astringent" means it reduces discharges. "Galactagogue" means it supports the production of breast milk. "Diuretic" means it increases the amount of water and salt expelled from the body as urine.)

Nettle is one of the most widely applicable plants we have. It strengthens and supports the whole body. It is one of the most powerful plants we have to deal with allergic rhinitis, more commonly known as pollen allergy or hay fever. Studies also show that it has a broad range of anti-inflammatory properties, so it is useful with migraines, arthritis, lupus pain, etc. It is an extremely nutritive plant, high in vitamins and minerals, particularly iron, silica, and potassium, and shows broad antifungal effects as well. Its diuretic effect promotes detoxification and works to prevent bladder infections. It also strengthens the kidneys and adrenals, an important function during pregnancy when those organs have an increased workload. The readily-assimilated high calcium content helps to diminish muscle pain in all areas of the body during pregnancy including the legs, round ligaments, cervix, back, and also during labor as well. With its high vitamin K content, it helps prevent excessive bleeding after birth. Because it strengthens the blood vessels and maintains arterial elasticity, it helps prevent hemorrhoids and varicose veins, which also helps to maintain a normal blood pressure.

Oat Straw:

Avena Sativa

Active Ingredients: 50% starch, proteins, alkaloids, saponins, flavones, sterols, Vitamin B, silica, & calcium, magnesium, silicon, potassium, & iron.

Actions: Nervine tonic, anti-depressant, nutritive, demulcent, vulnerary. ("Demulcent" means it soothes irritated tissue, and "vulnerary" means it aids in healing of wounds.)

Oat straw is one of the best remedies for "feeding" the nervous system. It is useful for combating exhaustion and depression; it strengthens the whole nervous system, making it a preventative and protective herb to enhance your ability to cope with stress. While being stimulating and energy-giving, it is also relaxing and an aid to sleep. Oat straw is also a uterine tonic, and works on strengthening the thyroid and balancing hormone production. It can be helpful for high blood pressure, varicose veins, and hemorrhoids. It is also a soother for the digestive tract. It also lowers blood sugar and is useful for fluid retention. It is one of the best sources for magnesium, which helps relieve irritability and enhance calcium absorption.

Red Raspberry Leaf (SW-p49):
Rubus idaeus

Active Ingredients: volatile oils, pectin, citric acid, malic acid, tannin, phosphorus, potassium, calcium, magnesium, & zinc, Vitamin A, B, C & E. Has the highest known herbal source of manganese.

Actions: Astringent, tonic, toning, pelvic and uterine relaxant.

Raspberry leaves have a long tradition of use in pregnancy to strengthen and tone the tissue of the womb, assisting contractions, and preventing excessive bleeding. Raspberry leaves also help tone the mucous membranes throughout the body, soothe the kidneys and urinary tract, and prevent excessive bleeding after the birth. Raspberry works on the digestive tract, stabilizing it. The benefits continue after birth as it helps milk production and recovery. The tonic and relaxant actions on the smooth muscles of the uterus act to reduce the pain of uterine contractions during childbirth and makes them more effective and productive, shortening the duration of labor.

NOTE: Raspberry leaf and nettle contain calcium in its most absorbable form. Spinach, chocolate, rhubarb, and brewer's yeast will interfere with the absorption of calcium. Also, calcium supplements made of bone meal and oyster shell should be avoided as they are not easily absorbed in the body and they have been shown to contain high levels of lead, mercury, cadmium, and other toxic metals.

Alfalfa:
Medicago sativa

Active Ingredients: vitamin K, iron, chlorophyll, vitamins A, B-6, E, D, & K, beta-carotene, biotin, folic acid, pantothenic acid, fatty acids, saponins, high in copper.

Actions: bitter, general tonic, alterative, diuretic.

Alfalfa has a history going back to ancient times, cherished for its nourishing abilities for people and animals. It has a deep tap root and grows in rich soils, making it very rich in trace minerals that it pulls up from deep below the surface. It purifies the blood and is a powerful tonic. It soothes the digestive tract, and contains the digestive enzyme betaine, and the saponins balance the intestinal flora.

Information compiled by Vickie Liguori of In Due Thyme Midwifery, 2006.

Other Dietary Deficiencies (SW-p49)

Avivia Romm, in her article "The Top Daily Supplements for Women," states:

> "A large 2009 study found 80% of Americans are low in virtually every color category of fruits and vegetables (leafy greens; red, orange, and yellow fruits and veggies; and the blue-purple varieties) leading to low-level nutritional deficiencies in plant-based vitamins, minerals, and phytochemicals (special plant-based chemicals that support detoxification and prevent inflammation). Yet we know from study after study that 80% of the chronic diseases we face

as we age are preventable with a healthy diet, particularly the nutrients we get from fruits and vegetables.

In 2009, the World Health Organization published a report stating that we have a nationwide magnesium deficiency—75 % of Americans consumed less magnesium than needed for optimum health. Low magnesium is associated with Type 2 diabetes, metabolic syndrome, elevated C-reactive protein (a major blood marker of inflammation), hypertension, atherosclerosis, migraine headache, and causes anxiety, sleep problems, depression, menstrual cramps, heart palpitations, chocolate cravings, and restless leg syndrome. Low magnesium is also a risk factor for Hashimoto's thyroiditis (a disorder that can lead to chronic inflammation of the thyroid and hypothyroidism). The statistics are grim on us getting adequate amounts of a number of other nutrients as well.

On top of this, the daily stressors that most of us face can, over time, take a toll on our health. I don't mean just the emotional kind of stress, though that can have an impact on your nutritional status, too. I mean the environmental kind, like toxins in our air, water, household products, cosmetics—pretty much everywhere—that require our bodies to work overtime detoxifying, which uses up a hefty dose of the phytonutrients and phytochemicals that help us detoxify and protect our cells from damage. Protective nutrients mean less inflammation, better elimination of environmental toxins, clearer thinking, more energy, and even slower aging!"

Aviva Romm also states:

"Based on several decades of research and practice in integrative women's health, these are the nutrients I often recommend to women as daily supplements. Unless otherwise specified, these are safe if you are on medications, pregnant, or nursing:

- A **multivitamin/multimineral supplement** to provide overall support and protection. Taking a daily multivitamin helps make sure you have the bases covered. I prefer Rainbow Light Women's One, which is whole-foods based, and only requires taking 1 pill daily. But any whole foods multi is usually a good bet. Go for non-GMO, organic, and free of dyes, additives, and colorings.

- **Vitamin D3**, for a total of 2000-4000 units daily. Vitamin D is responsible for hundreds of functions in the body, from healthy immunity to healthy bones. Vegetarians often ask me about a non-animal source. Unfortunately, I can't give you a definitive answer as to whether vitamin D2 or lichen-sourced D3 is as usable by the body as animal-based vitamin D3. Although you do get vitamin D from sun exposure, it may not be enough. It's best to get tested before supplementing so that you know how much you need. Ask your doctor to have your 25,OH-D level checked. An ideal test result should be between 40 and 80.

- **Magnesium**. I recommend glycinate unless there is constipation, and if there is, citrate often does the trick, for a daily total of 600 mg daily. Magnesium supports healthy bones, restful sleep, relaxed muscles, and balanced mood.

- **Fish oil**, 1-2 capsules daily. Omega-3 fats are important for reducing inflammation, maintaining heart health, improving mood, mind, and hair, and maintaining a healthy weight. An alternative source: DHA and/or EPA (plant-based Omega-3s). Vegans can take algae-sourced DHA, such as Life's DHA. Just keep in mind that DHA is not as easily converted to EPA, so you'll need to take a higher dose. Rejuvenation Science Labs has a vegan DHA and EPA supplement, which covers both bases, although I have not personally tried this brand.

- For vegans: **Vitamin B12** in a daily supplementation of 2.4 micrograms. This is especially important for vegans since B12 is not found in un-fortified, plant-based foods. If taking B12 orally, take it sublingually (under the tongue for quick absorption into the bloodstream). Make sure you choose a B12 in the form of methylcobalamin (check label), since this form of B12 is absorbed best."

Additional Herbs for Women's Health

There are other herbs that balance hormones and strengthen your female reproductive organs. Herbalist **Amanda Dilday** has put together this section for you to delve deeper into the plants that God has provided for our health as women. Please be discerning and do your own research. Speaking with a health care provider or herbalist will enable you to fine tune your exact needs as an individual.

NOTE: Some of the herbal guides in this section contain terms that may be unfamiliar. Here is a key to some of the vocabulary your audience may find most difficult:

- **Carminative:** relieves flatulence
- **Cardiotonic:** having a favorable effect on the action of the heart
- **Emmenagogue:** stimulates or increases menstrual flow
- **Nervine:** calming to the nerves
- **Diaphoretic:** induces perspiration
- **Analgesic:** pain relieving
- **Diuretic:** increases the passing of urine
- **Neoplastic:** can cause abnormal tissue growth (cysts, tumors, etc)
- **Hepatic:** relating to the liver
- **Alterative:** favorably alters the course of an ailment

Motherwort (SW-p52)
Leonorus cardiaca

Active ingredients: alkaloids, bitter glycosides, tannins, volatile oils, vitamin A

Actions: antispasmodic, aromatic, bitter, carminative, cardiotonic, emmenagogue, nervine, mild uterine stimulant, relaxant, sedative

Parts Used: flower and leaf

Motherwort has long been a friend and ally of women, especially mothers. This mother-herb not only has an affinity for the womb but also the heart. *Leonorus cardiaca*: the heart of a lion. What mother—what woman—does not need such a strong, brave heart as she walks through this world, witnessing its sorrows and carrying its burdens? To witness and to carry often causes us much anxiety, and for this, motherwort is strongly indicated. When our heart, full of care and worry, beats too quickly, a few drops of motherwort will bring comfort and quiet—a strong, steady rhythm. A heart tonic, nervine, and sedative, motherwort is indicated in cases of anxiety when symptoms include heart palpitations and panic attacks. A gentle emmenagogue, motherwort is useful when menses is delayed due to stress or anxiety.

Herbalist and author Matthew Wood says motherwort is indicated when a woman has "big, staring eyes". New mothers, mothers of young children, mothers of many children—we know that look, don't we? Hiding in the bathroom, we look in the mirror and see those big, staring eyes. Overwhelmed by all the busyness, messiness, responsibility, and crying, we need a moment to gather our thoughts—to quiet our hearts. We think we may never leave the bathroom, and then, a sweet little note is slipped under the door. Our hearts melt, and the tears come. And at this moment, when we are tense and confused by the overwhelming emotions that flood our mother-heart, herbalist Susun Weed thinks it's the perfect time for a few drops of motherwort. (I recommend keeping a small bottle of motherwort tincture in the medicine cabinet.)

Motherwort's bitter taste is a friend of the liver. Her bitterness stimulates the flow of bile and other digestive juices, promoting both digestion and absorption. By supporting the liver, motherwort contributes to balanced hormones—so necessary for healthy cycles, ready conception, and pleasant, steady moods. There is no question that she helps to ease anger and irritability.

Being quite bitter, motherwort is best used as a tincture. In a tea or infusion, she may be a little hard to swallow! Being a mild uterine stimulant, motherwort is not suggested for use in early pregnancy, but can be a great friend in the final weeks before the birth, helping the womb to find its rhythm and the heart its courage.

Lemon Balm (SW-p52)
Melissa officinalis

Active Ingredients: volatile oils, polyphenols, tannins, flavonoids

Actions: aromatic, antiviral, decongestant, carminative, antispasmodic, antidepressant, bitter tonic, nervine, relaxant, diaphoretic

Parts Used: leaf and flower

Lemon balm is herbal sunshine. Simply by her presence—by her fragrance—lemon balm is good medicine. Crush her leaves between your fingers, lift them to your nose, and breathe deeply. Her green goodness will rise to your head, bringing clarity and light, and reach into your heart, lifting its spirits and making it glad. Honestly, I'm not sure it's possible to smell lemon balm and not smile from the heart.

Lemon balm has an affinity for the digestive system, heart, and nervous system. A carminative, bitter, and antispasmodic, she encourages ease of digestion by relieving nausea, soothing upset stomachs, and improving poor appetites. Relieving tension, she may be used to relieve headaches, including migraines. Though sweet, her sour taste and bitter qualities stimulate both the liver and the gallbladder, enhancing both digestion and absorption. Cooling the liver, she aids in easing an angry and irritable spirit.

Lemon balm brings joy to the heart and soothes the nervous system. Lifting the spirit and quieting its worries, she gives relief to those suffering from excitable heart palpitations, panic attacks, and insomnia. When the heart is too excited, flitting and fluttering, lemon balm can calm it and ground it. In my experience, I have found lemon balm most helpful to those who are "high strung" or "easily excited". If someone's level of agitation or excitement makes *me* anxious and nervous, then I may slip them a cup of herbal sunshine.

A little side note: lemon balm is specifically indicated with sweaty palms. Often sweaty palms accompany nervousness and excitement. A diaphoretic, lemon balm can cool and release the heat while helping the body regulate fluids.

Lemon balm may be taken as a tincture or tea. An overnight infusion is refreshing.

Rose
Rose spp.

>Actions: astringent, relaxant, mild laxative, refrigerant, decongestant, nervine

>Active Ingredients: vitamin A, B, C, E, K, tannins, pectin, flavonoids, volatile oils, potassium, iron

>Parts used: leaf, petals, hips

Note: If harvesting your own roses, wild roses are best. But if cultivated roses are what is available to you, enjoy them! But be sure they have not been sprayed with pesticides.

Ah, rose. What a tender, comforting companion. She loves your heart and especially desires to offer her medicine when you are grieving. Very few herbs have the ability to touch the heart in as tender, yet powerful, a way as rose does. Often, when we are sad, or when we grieve, it is difficult for us to get a deep breath. Our hearts are closing in, tightening up, protecting themselves—and understandably so. But rose is able to come and help us open up and breathe again. Having soft petals and sharp thorns, she knows what it is to be tender yet protected. Let her teach you. In my experience, rose is especially comforting when we experience a miscarriage or stillbirth. She is a friend of the broken-hearted.

When my heart needs a tender, loving touch, I always go to rose. When the sadness rising up makes it difficult for me to breathe, I go to rose. When the heat of anger disturbs my grieving spirit, I go to rose to cool me. Rose is a plant deeply woven into the human story, and it is no wonder—she is a great gift to us.

You can enjoy the gift of rose in many ways. The petals and hips may be enjoyed as a tea or taken as a tincture. (Take note: rose petals are quite astringent. So, when making tea, a short steep may be best, or you can combine rose with other moistening herbs, like oats or marshmallow root, for a longer infusion and more balanced experience.) Rose petals can be used to make rose water or a divine rose-infused oil. You can sprinkle the petals into your bath. And the hips can be made into a nourishing jam. There are so many ways to interact with rose and receive her medicine. Experiment. Have fun. And let your heart lead you.

Chamomile
Matricaria chamomilla

> Active Ingredients: volatile oil, flavonoids, coumarins, choline, tannin, cyanogenic glycosides
>
> Actions: antispasmodic, bitter, carminative, relaxant, anti-inflammatory, analgesic, diuretic, diaphoretic, decongestant, antihistamine
>
> Parts used: flowers

Chamomile has an affinity for both the digestive system and nervous system. A relaxant and antispasmodic, she relieves tension, digestive upset—especially when caused by stress or tension, and headaches occasioned by the same. Often, when we don't feel well, we tend to complain and whine a bit more than usual, so chamomile is a wonderful ally when we need both relief from discomfort and a change of attitude. And those two things are so often needed just before our cycles. An antispasmodic and nervine relaxant, chamomile is an effective means of relieving premenstrual moodiness and cramps.

With its affinity for the digestive symptom, chamomile is a bitter, carminative, and antispasmodic, and so proves helpful in alleviating both nausea and morning sickness in early pregnancy.

Chamomile flowers may be enjoyed as a tea or a tincture—or even as a calming, infused oil. (Many times, I have rubbed chamomile onto my whiny little ones' hurting bellies.) Being quite bitter, chamomile is best steeped for only 10 or 15 minutes—any longer, and it's bitter taste will make it less pleasant to sip.

Most evenings, I enjoy a cup of chamomile tea. Often, there is a bit of honey and lavender in the mix, too. She relaxes me so I can let go of the day's busyness and fall asleep more easily.

Cleavers
Galium aparine

> Active Ingredients: gallotannic acid, citric acid, tannins, saponins, coumarin
>
> Actions: astringent, lymphatic, nervine, diuretic, alterative, anti-inflammatory, tonic, astringent, neoplastic
>
> Parts Used: aerial parts
>
> Note: *Best used fresh.* So full of moisture, cleavers does not dry well.

Every spring, cleavers reaches out her arms to grab us. She wants us to see her—use her—because she has deep, good medicine to offer us. After we have spent the winter sitting still and becoming sluggish, cleavers can help us do a bit of internal spring cleaning. She is a great friend of the lymphatic system—perhaps one of its dearest allies. Like an elegant chimney sweep, cleavers twirls and dances, removing debris and dislodging what is stuck. Enjoying her as a tea or tincture in early spring will keep our internal waters flowing clean.

Cleavers has a special affinity for swollen or painful lymph nodes under or behind the ears. Swollen tonsils can be cleansed and eased by her, and she is certainly indicated in cases of tonsillitis. With her affinity for the lymph, she is a strong ally of our breasts. She is powerful medicine in cases of fibrocystic breasts, or when there are cancers or tumors in the breast. In my own experience, cleavers is the go-to herb for mastitis. She quickly gets the lymph moving, and the milk flowing. Every new mother's postpartum supply basket should hold a tincture of fresh cleavers.

Cleavers loves our inner waters; she is a friend of the urinary system and the kidneys. Where there is fluid retention, edema, and bloating, she may be just what is needed to strengthen the kidneys in their work, and in so doing, get at the root of the excess water. A cooling diuretic with anti-inflammatory properties, she is useful with urinary tract infections (UTIs), cystitis, and other inflammations of the urinary system, and she is even useful in breaking up calcifications, such as kidney stones. Cleavers works deeply and with precision, getting at all those little particles that cause us irritation and pain.

Cleavers also has an affinity for our nervous system. She even physically resembles our nervous systems, with nerve endings, dendrites: lines of communication and connection. Her seeds even contain a bit of caffeine—which tells us she has medicine for our nerves. So, for those of us who are easily irritated by little things, who have all sorts of little-somethings that get under our skin, cleavers may be just the friend we need. She soothes the nerves, and helps us not be so tense—so aware and on guard—so ready to jump, or flinch, or react. She helps us be alert without being tense.

A specific indication for cleavers is overly sensitive skin, skin that itches and tickles and tingles easily.

Cleavers also has an affinity for the heart, especially for a heart that is tainted, or poisoned, by anger—especially if that anger is old and deep. Sometimes, anger can be so old and deep that we have forgotten it is there—are not even able to still feel it. If you suspect your heart, your inner waters, may run a little black with unforgiveness, or resentment, or even rage, perhaps cleavers could help you begin to be washed clean.

Red Clover
Trifolium pratense

> Active Ingredients: phenolic glycosides, flavonoids, coumarins, phytoestrogen, calcium, magnesium, potassium, Vitamin B complex, vitamin C, phosphorus, potassium, antioxidants (and that's just the beginning!)
>
> Actions: alterative, diuretic, antiviral, expectorant, antispasmodic, lymphatic
>
> Parts used: flowers

Red clover is a deeply nourishing tonic, even "supremely nourishing", according to herbalist Robin Rose Bennett. In agreement, herbalist Susun Weed points out that red clover's high vitamin content benefits the womb, her easily absorbed calcium and magnesium blesses the nervous system, and her high protein content benefits the entire body. Red clover's teacup overflows with nourishing minerals that are needed by every gland in the body, and so, she is a great restorer of hormone function. Alkalizing the body, she benefits the reproductive system by making the womb receptive to conception, and with all these nourishing qualities in mind, Susun Weed declares her "the single most useful herb in establishing fertility."

Red clover is especially indicated in cases of hard, even painful, lumps. In these cases, she has a special affinity for the neck.

Taken as a daily infusion or tincture, red clover is an herb that should be in every woman's apothecary. Here, I have only begun to speak of her rich medicine. So, I encourage you to read about her, gather her, and get to know her. She is a gift, nourishing us, cooling us, and gently (but effectively) reaching into our tenderest places.

Blue Vervain
Verbena hastata

> Active Ingredients: glycosides, alkaloid, bitter, volatile oils, tannin

> Actions: intense bitter, antispasmodic, diaphoretic, nervine, hepatic, sedative, astringent

> Parts used: aerial parts

Blue vervain is a precious gift to us, yet she is so little known. But if I could offer one herb to women, I believe it would be this one. Her medicine is rich and powerful, and life-saving. For me, blue vervain is the plant that saved my life, and I offer it to you with much love and many prayers for strength and healing.

Blue vervain is incredibly bitter—so bitter that it will send a shiver through your entire body—and this is a good thing. With her acrid taste, she wakes up, unfreezes, and reanimates the autonomic nervous system. In so doing, she not only relieves deep tension in the body, but also improves digestion, particularly the roles played by the liver and gallbladder. She restores the appetite.

Blue vervain is also a deep nervine tonic, antispasmodic, and sedative. Her ability to release tension in the body is extraordinary, and her skill is best seen when tension is held in the shoulders and the neck. She is so effective that she has traditionally been used for epilepsy and seizures, especially if the tremors begin in the neck. Herbalist Matthew Wood says that she is for "stiff-necked" people, a state that can describe us not only physically but also constitutionally. Are we being stubborn? Pressing forward when we should step back? Deciding it's "our way or the highway"? If so, we likely need a few drops of blue vervain.

Blue vervain is necessary for those who have high standards but are not able to reach them. Often, this is because the standards are not reasonable. The goal may be good and honorable (or not), but it may not be the season for it—the strength and resources might not be there. And this is another indicator for blue vervain: if someone is "strong above but weak below". They have wonderful ideas (ideals) and much passion, but they do not have the stamina to finish the job. Physically, this can be seen when someone is mentally strong but has a weak digestive and reproductive system.

Blue vervain is a friend to women in other ways. She is especially helpful when women experience crazy food cravings and binges before and during the menstrual cycle. Herbalist Matthew Wood, and others, say this is likely due to an excess of progesterone during this time. He says a woman may feel "driven to eat" and then not eat much else the rest of the month. Blue vervain is also useful when there are heavy cycles and menstrual cramps, and she is strongly indicated when anger—strong, raging anger—is part of the premenstrual picture. She gets that liver moving, relieves pent-up tension, and so, helps be a little less irritable and bit more patient.

With all my heart, I believe every woman should have blue vervain growing in her flower bed. We carry so much, we do so much, we expect so much—and so, we need so much. With open, thankful hands, receive the gift offered in blue vervain.

Alternative Therapies for Cycle Health

I wanted to include more than just herbs for alternative ways to better your health surrounding your cycle, so here I have provided suggestions for a variety of beneficial tools and practices, with the hope that you and your class will pick and choose which work for your lifestyle and budget.

Essential Oils

I use oils in everyday life with my clients and family as an alternative to running to the doctor for minor colds and illnesses, and also for growing pains, rashes, or muscle discomfort. There are so many uses for oils! I wanted to include a section about them, specifically geared toward menstruation. I asked my friend to give us her expertise and knowledge concerning which ones would be good to look into for cycle health. Here is what my friend, Certified Holistic Health Coach Shana Evans, has supplied:

"Many women have great success with using essential oils for hormone balance and to alleviate cramping, PMS and other symptoms. In many cases, using an essential oils safely (topically and diluted) can help alleviate the struggles of PMS and even helping hormones balance over time. Essential oils can be very powerful and effective when used correctly.

Here are just a few suggestions:

1. Dragon Time

This blend may help with easing PMS symptoms and menstrual discomforts associated with the normal menstrual cycle. Mood swings and tension, and even mild cramping, may be due to the hormonal shifts that women may experience. Dragon Time can help promote feelings of stability and calmness during cycles of moodiness and even help to restore emotional balance.

This blend contains 6 essential oils including:

- **Fennel** helps support digestion

- **Clary Sage** is supportive to female hormones

- **Marjoram** is supportive to the musculoskeletal system and nerves. Helps to ease discomforts of periods

- **Lavender** is relaxing and may help with anxiousness, PMS symptoms, and head tension associated with menstruation

- **Blue Yarrow** is supportive to hormone balance

- **Jasmine** helps to combat moodiness, including crabbiness and sadness associated with menstrual cycle changes

Dragon Time can be diluted 50:50 with your carrier oil of choice and applied topically where desired. Some areas of comfort may include temples, lower abdomen, and lower back.

(**Carrier oil**, also known as base oil, is used to dilute essential oils and absolutes before they are applied to the skin in massage and aromatherapy. It can be almond oil, olive oil, or fractionated coconut oil.)

You can also dilute for a full body massage. Apply over lower abdomen and apply a warm compress. You may also apply over the inside and outside of the ankle area, which is the ovary VitaFlex point. Dragon Time blend can also be diffused.

(**VitaFlex points** are places on the body that practitioners believe align with other parts of the body and can be influenced by essential oils, massage, etc.)

NOTE: Dragon Time Can cause sun sensitivity, use precaution with application.

Monthly Roll-On Recipe:
For that extra support surrounding PMS and the menstruation part of the menstrual cycle: in a 10-mL glass roller top bottle, add 2 drops Helichrysum, 10 drops Geranium, 10 drops Cypress and 3 drops Peppermint. Top with a carrier oil such as Young Living's V-6 or fractionated coconut oil. Shake gently before application. Use along with Dragon Time blend for extra support, if needed.

2. Clary Sage
Women around the world praise clary sage for its ability to get them through that difficult week every month.

Clary sage may help relieve bloating, mood swings, compulsive eating, and other PMS woes through simply inhaling the oil. You can use a diffuser, or simply soak a cotton ball and place by your bedside. A steam facial is also a great way to relax and get rid of the PMS blues.

For menstrual cramps, use 10ml of a carrier oil and a few drops of clary sage essential oil. Rub your abdomen gently with the mixture for several minutes. A warm, soothing bath with the diluted clary sage mixture is also a great way to help relieve cramping.

3. FemiGen Supplement

FemiGen capsules were formulated with herbs and amino acids designed to balance and support the female reproductive system from youth through menopause. FemiGen combines whole food herbs like wild yam, damiana, and dong quai, along with synergistic amino acids and select essential oils to supply nutrition that is supportive of the special needs of the female systems.

How to Use: Take 2 capsules with breakfast and 2 capsules with lunch.

Ingredients:

- Magnesium
- Damiana (*Turnera diffusa*) leaf
- *Epimedium sagittatum* aerial plant
- Wild Yam (*Dioscorea villosa*) root
- Dong Quai (*Angelica sinensis*) root
- Muira Puama (*Ptychopetalum olacoides*) root
- Ginseng (*Panax quinquefolium*) root
- Licorice (*Glycyrrhiza glabra*) root extract
- Black Cohosh (*Cimicifuga racemosa*) root
- L-carnitine
- Dimethylglycine HCl
- Cramp Bark (*Viburnum opulus*) bark
- Squaw Vine (*Mitchella repens*) aerial parts
- L-phenylalanine
- L-cystine
- L-cysteine HCl
- Fennel (*Foeniculum vulgare*) seed
- Clary Sage (*Salvia sclarea*) flowering top
- Sage (*Salvia officinalis*) leaf
- Ylang Ylang (*Cananga odorata*) flower

Please visit www.seedtoseal.com for a better understanding of why ONLY Young Living Essential Oils are recommended.

NOTE: If you would like to discuss further, please contact:

Shana Evans, Certified Holistic Health Coach
Phone: 540-533-2090
Email: ylcoachshana@gmail.com
Website: www.yldailydrops.com

Massage

Massage throughout the month, or even once a month, is so edifying for your body, bringing life and flow to your cardiovascular system and lymphatic system. Benefits include less discomfort, less bleeding, less cramping, and fewer mood swings. It helps to increase relaxation, which can help relieve the tension in your body that can cause more discomfort during your cycle.

> "A recent study by the University of Miami Medical School of women with severe Premenstrual Syndrome (PMS) divided them into a massage therapy group and a progressive muscle relaxation therapy group.
>
> The women receiving massage showed a decrease in anxiety, depression, and perceived pain, as well as other PMS symptoms. 'Overall,' the study concluded, 'massage therapy may be an effective long-term aid for pain reduction and water retention, and short-term for decreasing anxiety and improving mood for women with...PMS.'"—from "The Benefits of Massage During Menstruation," www.massageenvy.com

Just with any other alternative health help, there can be disadvantages. Doing all things in moderation and keeping everything in balance is the key. Please speak with a healthcare provider if you have any doubts or questions concerning any of these therapies.

> "Keep in mind…Although massage can aid in fighting off the menstrual pain, it does increase blood flow which means a massage may increase your menstrual flow for a day after the massage; keep in mind, however, the increase in blood flow also has positive effects on menstruation. Increased blood flow may reduce cramps and back pain." — Can You Get a Message While on Your Period? (Pub. January 18th, 2017)

Chiropractic Care

Celeste Krawchuk (Berryville Chiropractic) offers this overview of chiropractic care:

> "Chiropractic is a natural (drug- and surgery-free) form of healthcare that is based on keeping your nervous system functioning at its best. This allows the rest of your body to be as healthy as possible.
>
> Chiropractic adjustments are safe, painless, and fairly quick. Adjustments are what a chiropractor does to make sure each vertebra in your spine is lined up and moving properly. Sometimes, you will hear a "popping" sound like cracking your knuckles, other times the chiropractor will use an adjusting tool, such as an activator, and you will not hear that sound.

Chiropractic care helps decrease the symptoms of PMS and other discomforts associated with menstruation, especially cramping, lower back pain, headaches (including migraines), and breast tenderness. This is done by adjusting any misalignments found in the spine. The most common areas of the spine that affect menstruation and its associated symptoms are in the lower back, sacrum, and upper neck

Keeping your nervous system working as well as possible allows your endocrine system (hormones) to become better regulated. By affecting the endocrine system, chiropractic care helps keep your cycle regular (around 28 days). The area of the spine that most affects your endocrine system is the upper neck.

Seeing a Chiropractor will help your body better manage the changes it will be going through during early womanhood and beyond."

Source: www.berryvillechiropractic.com

Acupuncture

"Chinese Medicine offers effective support for women to get to the root of hormonal issues. We support women throughout the cycle with acupuncture and herbs to help restore hormonal balance. Many women will see a positive shift in the health of their cycles in three to four months of regular treatments." —Daniela Freda, "Four Signs of a Healthy Menstrual Cycle That All Women Should Know"

I have used acupuncture for healing in the past for vertigo, hip and pelvic pain, and for post-cancer healing. I am always amazed at how beneficial and effective it is. Colleen Porter has been treating me. I asked her to share with you how acupuncture works and is a great "help" for cycle health:

"In traditional Chinese medicine, we believe that your body is made up of pathways of energy called "channels" and through the channels flows something called "qi" (pronounced "chee"). Qi is your life force energy, like the spark that animates a living thing. In order for you to be ideally healthy and well, you need to have qi moving in a constant flow through your body, in the right quantity and moving without blockage. The qi moves blood through your body creating proper circulation and nourishment to all your tissues.

At different times of your menstrual cycle, the qi and blood should be moving into particular channels. Before your period, as your body moves toward ovulation, qi and blood need to be nourished to replenish the qi and blood lost during your menstrual cycle and to encourage the growth of a new egg. During ovulation, it is necessary to have a calm spirit and proper qi flow to your liver in order to comfortably and easily ovulate. And then after ovulation, it is extra important to keep your body active and moving to encourage blood and qi flow to the uterus as you prepare for a period.

Diet, activity level, emotional health, and proper sleep can all affect the flow of qi and blood at any stage of the cycle. It is important to get extra rest and good nutrition when your body needs it and to make sure to get enough exercise and stress relief when that is called for.

Acupuncture and Chinese herbal medicine are some ways to help balance the stages of your cycle when you're having trouble ovulating, having irregular periods, dramatic emotional changes with your cycles, or having difficult periods." —Colleen Porter, Licensed Acupuncturist

Yoga or Other Movement & Stretching (SW-p62)

As a yoga instructor, I am going to mention the benefits of yoga. If you do not believe in the spiritual discipline of yoga or you are concerned with the safety of practicing due to Christian convictions, I urge you to explore how yoga is not a religion, but rather is a way we can bring breath, movement, and stretching to our daily lives. Words like "mindfulness" and "meditation" have been correlated with one religion or worldview, but we as Christians know that we see the words "meditation" and "sober-minded" in the very Word of God. (Please visit the Holy Yoga website: **holyyoga.net** for more information regarding Christianity and yoga practice.)

> *The Message* Bible says it this way:
> There's more: God's Word warns us of danger
> and directs us to hidden treasure.
> Otherwise how will we find our way?
> Or know when we play the fool?
> Clean the slate, God, so we can start the day fresh!
> Keep me from stupid sins,
> from thinking I can take over your work;
> Then I can start this day sun-washed,
> scrubbed clean of the grime of sin.
> These are the words in my mouth;
> these are what I chew on and pray.
> Accept them when I place them
> on the morning altar,
> O God, my Altar-Rock,
> God, Priest-of-My-Altar.
> **Psalm 19:11-14**

And…

> Summing it all up, friends, I'd say you'll do best by filling your minds and meditating on things true, noble, reputable, authentic, compelling, gracious—the best, not the worst; the beautiful, not the ugly; things to praise, not things to curse. Put into practice what you learned from me, what you heard and saw and realized. Do that, and God, who makes everything work together, will work you into his most excellent harmonies. - **Philippians 4:8-9**

> "We know that yoga is a spiritual discipline much like fasting, meditation, and prayer that cannot be owned by one specific religion. While yoga predates Hinduism, Hindus were the first to give yoga a written structure. Yoga postures were originally named in Sanskrit." — Holyyoga.net, "What We Believe"

Doing yoga regularly will improve mood, strength, and help you be spiritually ready for the challenges you may face during your actual period. However, avoiding extensive inversions during your cycle is wise; we do not want the blood flow to be "going against the tide," so to speak.

> "We know that yoga is a spiritual discipline much like fasting, meditation, and prayer that cannot be owned by one specific religion. While yoga predates Hinduism, Hindus were the first to give yoga a written structure. Yoga postures were originally named in Sanskrit."— Holyyoga.net, "What We Believe"

Hydration

Water is the best source for your daily fluid needs. Tea can provide the same hydration and benefits as water as long as it is not caffeinated. You will want to choose organic herbs and supplements when possible to avoid risks associated with pesticides and chemicals. Sports drinks are not as beneficial as your own homemade version using less sugar. Here is a recipe to make a healthier version at home:

Lemon Energy Aide

4 cups filtered water

1/2 cup freshly squeezed lemon juice

1/4 teaspoon celtic sea salt or real salt

1/4 cup raw honey (or more to taste)

a few drops of concentrated mineral drops (optional)

a few drops of Rescue Remedy (optional)

Daily Exercise & Stretching

Our bodies were created to be moving. Some type of exercise should be implemented daily as a means for better health. There are various forms of exercise and you will need to explore and seek out the one that best fits your preference, needs, and schedule. Movement in our bodies keep the internal systems running smoothly; digestive, respiratory, lymphatic, and circulatory health is vital to our overall well-being.

> "The God who made the world and everything in it, this Master of sky and land, doesn't live in custom-made shrines or need the human race to run errands for him, as if he couldn't take care of himself. He makes the creatures; the creatures don't make him. Starting from scratch, he made the entire human race and made the earth hospitable, with plenty of time and space for living so we could seek after God, and not just grope around in the dark but actually *find* him. He doesn't play hide-and-seek with us. He's not remote; he's *near*. **We live and move in him,** can't get away from him! One of your poets said it well: 'We're the God-created.' Well, if we are the God-created, it doesn't make a lot of sense to think we could hire a sculptor to chisel a god out of stone for *us*, does it?" - **Acts 17:24-29**

Types of exercise to include in your daily schedules (SW-p64):

- Stretching & postures through Holy Yoga or other means of whole body stretching
- Walking - in the evening to help digest food and allow you to sleep deeper and more soundly
- Aerobics - high or low impact
- Weight lifting - gentle or advanced, combined with appropriate diet to maintain balance
- Sports - try different ones and find a good match for you
- Dance - worship, lyrical, upbeat, square, contra - so many to choose from

ACTIVITY: What works for you? (SW-p64)

- Have the class discuss what type of exercise works for them and why it works.
- What has not worked, and why has it not fit you or your schedule?
- How can you balance work, play, and daily routines?
- When is best to fit in your daily exercise? Morning? Evening?

Have the class stand up and stretch their arms above their heads—to the left, to the right, to center, and help them connect their breath to their movement.

- Inhale; reach arms high above head, spread fingers wide, keep shoulders down
- Exhale as you tilt body to the left (moon shape)
- Inhale; come back center
- Exhale; go to right, leaning toward right body
- Inhale; center
- Exhale; back bend slightly from upper body
- Inhale; center

Discuss how that made them feel; do they feel energized, more focused, alert, etc.?

<h1 style="text-align:center">Chapter 8
TAKING RESPONSIBILITY</h1>

REVIEW (SW-p66)

- What herbs might be good for calming your anxious spirit?

- What do you do for your health as far as diet, nutrition or exercise?

As women, we would benefit from learning and understanding the way our bodies are created and how we can obtain optimal health of our bodies. This means not transferring our responsibility to others through ignorance. (The word "ignorance" means lack of knowledge on a particular subject.) We may have stumbled in this area in the past, but we do better when we know better. Future generations can then be women *embracing* God's design with all humility and thankfulness!

ACTIVITY: Role Playing

Have the students and mother/mentors role play different situations in regards to how they can take responsibility for their health. Situations where having more information would be helpful and edifying, than situations where not having information and knowledge would be more difficult. How is your decision making affected by the knowledge you have or don't have?

We must exercise caution as we research and obtain information about our cycles and menstruation. Always check with your mother before googling or searching for subject matter. This is for your protection and also to keep the lines of communication open with your mother or family members you trust.

> "We need to take responsibility for our bodies and our cycles. We need to research and know how they work and why they work this way. What are the ramifications of this design and how does it affect me? How can I teach a positive aspect of this design to my daughters? We need to see the importance of using these seasons as opportunities to teach about God's goodness and mercy and faithfulness to us as women. There are so many significant aspects of each cycle and I think you will be truly amazed to learn about them. The learning process is "owning it", and also understanding that we are not to be ignorant on how God has designed our bodies. He tells us to get wisdom and to understand. The scriptures are full of exhortations to get knowledge and wisdom. Why would our cycles and how they work be any different? God can be revealed in all things, even in our cycles. This is truly amazing!"
> –Doran Richards

Knowledge and Wisdom

Be careful; there is a lot of knowledge to be had in our culture, and you must not fall into a trap of getting false knowledge. First and foremost, we should seek out Godly knowledge and understanding, which leads to wisdom. Where is our one source of Truth? The Bible, God's Word.

Here are some scriptures that speak on the importance of getting knowledge and understanding:

Proverbs 2:6 - And here's why: God gives out wisdom free, is plain-spoken in knowledge and Understanding. He's a rich mine of common sense for those who live well, a personal bodyguard to the candid and sincere. He keeps his eye on all who live honestly, and pays special attention to his loyally committed ones.

Proverbs 1:7 - Start with God—the first step in learning is bowing down to God; only fools thumb their noses at such wisdom and learning.

Proverbs 2:10,11 - So now you can pick out what's true and fair, find all the good trails! Lady Wisdom will be your close friend, and Brother Knowledge your pleasant companion. Good Sense will scout ahead for danger, insight will keep an eye out for you. They'll keep you from making wrong turns, or following the bad direction, of those who are lost themselves and can't tell a trail from a tumbleweed. These losers who make a game of evil and throw parties to celebrate perversity, traveling paths that go nowhere, wandering in a maze of detours and dead ends.

(SW-p67) All true knowledge is from God. His word is sufficient for our needs. Let us always look to it in prayer for answers concerning life and our monthly cycles.

"There is a ton of misinformation out there, so just make sure you do the research so you don't fall into the trap that so many parents in our culture have fallen into…blindly following the cultural trends. These trends are often unhealthy for families and can be especially detrimental to children. Some common beliefs are just simply false information! Only you can decide what is right for you and your family…so in order to make an informed decision, you have to do the research." —Tina Smith, www.fresnofamily.com

God tells us not to follow trends in our culture. Not to "go along" with what everyone else is doing *because* it is what everyone is doing. Instead, we are to be set apart.

Romans 12:2 - So here's what I want you to do, God helping you: Take your everyday, ordinary life—your sleeping, eating, going-to-work, and walking-around life—and place it before God as an offering. Embracing what God does for you is the best thing you can do for him. Don't become so well-adjusted to your culture that you fit into it without even thinking. Instead, fix your attention on God. You'll be changed from the inside out. Readily recognize what he wants from you, and quickly respond to it. Unlike the culture around you, always dragging you down to its level of immaturity, God brings the best out of you, develops well-formed maturity in you.

Colossians 2:8 - Watch out for people who try to dazzle you with big words and intellectual double-talk. They want to drag you off into endless arguments that never amount to anything. They spread their ideas through the empty traditions of human beings and the empty superstitions of spirit beings. But that's not the way of Christ. Everything of God gets expressed in him, so you can see and hear him clearly. You don't need a telescope, a microscope, or a horoscope to realize the fullness of Christ, and the emptiness of the universe without him. When you come to him, that fullness comes together for you, too. His power extends over everything.

"When we obtain knowledge, we have to make sure not to shove it down someone else's throat. We all have different walks with God; we are all at different stages and maturity levels. Where I may be in my understanding is not where you might be in yours. Let us walk in grace, encouraging one another to get knowledge, understanding and wisdom about our cycle and phases of womanhood, yet doing it with a spirit of love, uplifting and mentoring in our hearts, in a Godly manner! That is what will speak mountains to our friends and family as well as the culture around us." —Doran Richards

(SW-p68) I want to introduce you to a concept about education that comes from Classical antiquity. The Classical model of education is based on a concept that can carry over to all issues in life and how we obtain education for any particular subject. Let us explore this concept just a bit and you too will see how it makes sense in the area of our first cycle beginning our womanhood. I found this to be fascinating and true:

The classical model uses three stages of learning:

> **Grammar**
>
> **Dialectic (or Logic)**
>
> **Rhetoric**

According to scripture, the same terms would be:

> **Knowledge**
>
> **Understanding**
>
> **Wisdom**

In other words, to learn something new (in this case, about menstruation) you must:

> Input the vocabulary and basic rules and patterns associated with the concept— **KNOWLEDGE**
>
> Process the new information so that you personally understand it—**DIALECTIC**
>
> And then do something with it to demonstrate mastery—**RHETORIC**

Taking responsibility means that we need to have an active role in understanding our cycle health. This means getting understanding, which means gaining knowledge on the particular subject or issue surrounding us at any given season in our lives—it is no different for how we become woman by starting our cycle!

Proverbs 4:4-9 - Never walk away from wisdom—she guards your life; love her—she keeps her eye on you. Above all and before all, do this: Get wisdom! Write this at the top of your list: Get understanding! Throw your arms around her—believe me, you won't regret it; never let her go—she'll make your life glorious. She'll garland your life with grace, she'll festoon your days with beauty.

You can discuss this with your class and, if you have time, you can highlight this information about scripture knowledge and its importance. This is one more way we can be examples of Christ, to know the Word and seek the Word's wisdom.

Scripture Knowledge

by Pastor Jose B. Cabajar

"Knowledge is an asset that produces multiple advantages and benefits to be enjoyed by the possessor. Getting knowledge is a natural process; it starts the moment a child is born. Attitude towards learning affects the measure of knowledge that will be earned by a person. A good attitude gives the student a good way to gain more knowledge. A bad attitude not only blocks the progress of one's education, but also leads him to ignorance and other unpleasant consequences.

(SW-p69) A person who rejects knowledge is not considered a sound person, but a man who embraces knowledge will become successful in his chosen course. Knowledge comes before understanding, understanding comes before wisdom and fear of God comes before sound wisdom. Gaining the right knowledge is the key to a better understanding and having the right understanding leads a man to the gate of wisdom.

Scripture knowledge is the best knowledge every living man could gain. This kind of treasure cannot be compared with silver and gold. It surpasses the riches of the whole world and that is the reason why the world cannot afford to give it. It has been said that no man can find his way to God without the Word of God.

The Word of God is powerful. Living by the Word produces strong faith and godly living. The Word of God should not be a light thing in a corner, but a wonderful treasure one should be proud of. Well-lived Word of God glorifies God, but well-displayed head knowledge without application will push a man to his own spiritual shipwreck…

…Well-lived spiritual knowledge glorifies God. May our God-given knowledge be a precious part of our lives as we serve the Lord Jesus Christ."

Here are some more scriptures dealing with **knowledge, understanding,** and **wisdom** – allowing us to see, as we read, the impact this has toward our health:

Proverbs 5:1-2 - Dear friend, pay close attention to this, my wisdom; listen very closely to the way I see it. Then you'll acquire a taste for good sense; what I tell you will keep you out of trouble.

Proverbs 18:15 - Wise men and women are always learning, always listening for fresh insights.

Proverbs 19:8 - Grow a wise heart—you'll do yourself a favor; keep a clear head—you'll find a good life.

Our knowledge is not just for mere knowing for our own benefit, but please know how important it is that we glorify God with any and all knowledge we obtain. What is the chief end of man? To glorify our Father in heaven and enjoy Him forever. And we are to know God, and to make Him known.

Chapter 9
ABNORMALITIES & OTHER CYCLE CONSIDERATIONS

REVIEW (SW-p70)

- Why is it important that we seek knowledge about our monthly cycle health?

- Is all information available to us—on internet and in the media—good information?

You will see, throughout this course, areas of concern or interest that are not covered in depth. The purpose of this chapter is to help you know there are more issues surrounding menses and menstruation about which you may want to research and gain knowledge.

Some of these topics may come up during the course as questions from your students or their mothers. Always try to provide them with general information and let them find their own answers for a particular subject. It is important that everyone follow their own beliefs, especially when it comes to intimate topics such as menses.

This chapter is designed to stimulate further research into menstruation for you and your daughter/class. Always consult your own health care professional, midwife, or herbalist if you have any questions regarding your or your daughter's cycle.

As the teacher of this course, you are at liberty to use the information found here or leave it out entirely. Be aware of your biases and personal opinions when presenting this information to the students and mothers in the class. Let them form their own beliefs based on factual information for them individually. We pray that this course will help to enable everyone to have confidence and assurance during this season in their lives.

Amenorrhea (amen·or·rhea)

Amenorrhea is a menstrual disorder characterized by the absence of menstrual periods. It is a condition that affects 2-5% of women in North America. Women who are pregnant or going through menopause naturally have amenorrhea, but for young girls and women in their childbearing years, it is not normal. It can be particularly worrisome because it is an indicator of a health problem.

Amenorrhea is classified into two types:

Primary Amenorrhea: This occurs when a girl hasn't gotten her period by age 16. Most girls hit puberty around age 11 or 12, which causes an increase in hormones, stimulating the body to produce a period. Girls with primary amenorrhea may not have enough of these hormones in their bodies to begin menstruating. Primary amenorrhea is common among girls who are below the healthy weight threshold for their height or highly athletic, because they do not have enough fat to help produce the necessary hormones.

Secondary Amenorrhea: Women with secondary amenorrhea at one point experienced normal periods. Then, for some reason, their periods stopped. In order to be considered to have secondary amenorrhea (medically), your periods must have stopped for at least three months. It is usually the result of reproductive problems or hormonal complications. Stress and sudden, excessive weight loss can contribute to this as well.

Both primary and secondary amenorrhea require a visit to a physician or hormone specialist.

Causes of Amenorrhea
Most women get their periods every 28-35 days. Of course, there will be some fluctuation in any young girl's monthly cycles, especially if she has just begun to menstruate. Absence of a period for more than 3 months, especially after establishing a predictable monthly pattern, justifies a visit to the Health Care Provider.

(SW-68) Your menstrual cycle is actually quite responsive to environmental triggers. Poor nutrition and stress can wreak havoc on your period. If a person has amenorrhea, it is likely that something has caused her hormone levels to fall out of sync. As a result, her body is no longer producing a period. Factors that can contribute to hormonal problems include:

- improper nutrition

- strenuous exercise

- rapid weight loss or gain

- disordered eating, anorexia, or bulimia

- stress

- problems with your pituitary gland, hypothalamus, or ovaries

Complications of Amenorrhea
Amenorrhea is not a condition to be taken lightly. If you have noticed that your periods have stopped, it is important to find out why so that you can try to restore your cycle.

Treatment of Amenorrhea
There are natural, effective treatments for amenorrhea, which should help to restore your periods. Ask your healthcare provider, acupuncturist, chiropractor, midwife, or herbalist what they recommend for treatments.

NOTE: For more information on amenorrhea, see www.epigee.org/menstruation/amenorrhea.html. This site was written, researched, and published to the web by Monnica Williams, MA., who has spent over 15 years counseling and assisting women in crisis.

Dysmenorrhea (dys·men·or·rhea)

Dysmenorrhea refers to the pain or discomfort that comes with menstruation, namely cramps.

Other symptoms may include: headache, diarrhea, constipation, urinary frequency, and fainting. Although not a serious medical problem, dysmenorrhea usually describes a woman with menstrual symptoms severe enough to keep her from functioning for a day or more.

Most teens do not suffer from dysmenorrhea because their uterus is still growing. As they mature, they may experience painful periods. Symptoms may begin one to two days before menses, peak on the first day of flow, and subside during that day or over several days. The pain is typically described as a dull aching or cramping and often radiates to the lower back. The pain is thought to be contractions of the uterus, caused by an overabundance of prostaglandins (a hormone-like substance normally found in your body). Prostaglandins are known to stimulate uterine contractions.

There are many over-the-counter pain relievers that may provide help, such as ibuprofen or naproxen sodium. A heating pad works well for cramps when used with over the counter pain medications. Adhesive, self-heating thermal patches (which generally stay warm for 8 hours) are nice to use as well, especially since they fit well under clothing and don't inhibit movement like electric heating pads. Herbal remedies also exist that can relieve symptoms. Some women benefit from exercise, some from rest.

It is important to rule out medical conditions that may be causing dysmenorrhea. Endometriosis or fibroids are examples of possible underlying conditions. Some methods of birth control can also stimulate stronger contractions, causing cramping. It is important that a healthcare provider is consulted when you suspect dysmenorrhea.

For more information on dysmenorrhea, see:

www.coolnurse.com/dysmenorrhea.htm
http://womenshealth.about.com/cs/crampsmenstrual/a/cramps.htm
www.ehow.com/how_1960_relieve-menstrual-cramps.html

Menorrhagia (men·or·rha·gia)

Menorrhagia is abnormal uterine bleeding, or vaginal bleeding that is different from normal menstrual periods. It includes very heavy bleeding or unusually long periods, periods too close together, and bleeding between periods. Other causes of abnormal bleeding include uterine fibroids and polyps. Treatment for abnormal bleeding depends on the cause as determined by a healthcare professional.

Endometriosis (en·do·me·tri·osis) (SW-72)

With this condition, tissue normally found only in the uterus starts to grow outside the uterus—in the ovaries, fallopian tubes, or other parts of the pelvic cavity. It can cause abnormal bleeding, dysmenorrhea, and general pelvic pain.

Warnings for Menstruation

What happens if you don't see regular monthly cycles? Or you feel like the bleeding time is long and out of the norm for your daughter's age group? We have some guidelines for you to consider. Consult a medical professional if you or your daughter experience any of these menstrual symptoms/ conditions:

- No menstrual period within three years of breast development.
- No menstrual period by age 13, with no signs of pubertal development.
- No menstrual period by 14, with signs of excess facial or body hair (hirsutism).
- No menstrual period by 14, with a history or examination suggestive of excessive exercise or an eating disorder.
- No menstrual period by 14, with concerns about genital tract problems.
- No menstrual flow by 15.
- Menstrual periods that become "markedly irregular" after happening regularly every month.
- Menstrual periods occurring more than every 21 days.
- Menstrual periods occurring less than every 45 days.
- Menstrual periods occurring 90 days apart, even for one cycle.
- Menstrual periods that last more than seven days.
- Menstrual periods requiring frequent pad / tampon changes (more than once every one or two hours).

ACTIVITY: Abnormalities (SW-p73)

Have the girls review by writing the 4 big words we just discussed. In their workbooks they will have this:

List the four abnormalities we just discussed.

Hygiene and Self-Care

Shaving

When girls begin their menses, one corresponding issue is body hair and shaving areas like the underarms and legs. This is a topic for each mother and daughter to discuss when they feel the time is right. This will vary for many young girls and their mothers may have a difference of opinion on what age is appropriate to begin shaving.

When a young lady is ready, the following information may be helpful:

> The American Academy of Pediatrics says: "You may [also] notice hair under your arms and on your legs. Many women shave this hair. There is no medical reason to shave, it is simply a personal choice. If you decide to shave, be sure to use a lot of soap and water and a clean razor made for women. It is a good idea to use your own personal razor or electric shaver and not to share one with your family or friends."

Girls need a shaving tool that is gentle to their sensitive skin. It takes lots of practice to use a razor. Having adult supervision as a young girl is learning to shave and discussion about this topic is essential. Moms: make sure you keep that communication level open and check in with your girls often!

Basic Instructions:

- Shave in a warm shower or bath, if possible.

- Wait a few minutes before starting in order to let the leg hair soften. If you take showers, wait until the end of the shower to shave.

- Sit on the ledge in your shower, if possible. If your shower has no place to sit, raise one leg against the wall of the shower and balance carefully.

- Apply a small amount of shaving or moisturizing cream, rubbing it into a thick lather and spreading it over your leg. Soap has a tendency to dry out your skin.

- Place the razor at the base of your ankle and gently pull the razor up your leg, working in sections (and rinsing in between strokes) until your entire leg is shaved. If you experience razor burn, try shaving in the same direction as the hair growth (down). You may not get as clean a shave, but you'll avoid those little red bumps.

- Rinse.

- Repeat for the other leg.

- Pat dry and moisturize.

There are products available that aren't so abrasive to the skin or that can or may cause rash due to the slippery stripe they put at the top of a lot of razors. There are companies that sell razors that have more natural components like charcoal in the strip at top for lubrication. One company is called Billie who claim on their website, "Our 5-blade razor is encased in charcoal shave soap for an incredibly smooth glide every time. Bonus: it comes with a magic holder to keep your razor stored safely on your shower wall.

Tips for Beginner Shaver (SW-p74)

- You can use moisturizing cream instead of shaving cream. It is kinder to the skin than shaving cream when your legs or underarms are dry.

- Go slowly, taking your time. Use the razor in the same direction as the hair growth to avoid cuts and ingrown hairs.

- Shaving in the shower is good because the hair is softer when wet and warm. (Don't use an electric shaver in the shower!)

- Rinse the razor often while shaving to get rid of the hair. Change the blade often, before it gets blunt—a blade that isn't sharp is more likely to catch the skin and cause a nick.

- Using a moisturizing cream or coconut oil after shaving will soothe the skin.

Cleanliness

Personal hygiene means personal cleanliness. During menstruation, there is an increase in the production of oil by our body. We also perspire more heavily so we must give special attention to our personal cleanliness before and during menstruation. This will add to our comfort and confidence.

While we briefly discussed cleanliness and hygiene in **Chapter 5** when we went over bodily changes, here are several tips to help maintain cleanliness during this delicate period:

- Take a bath or shower daily, especially during this time. Make sure to gently wash your labia and vaginal area to get rid of odor and germs.

- To avoid underarm odor, apply deodorant to your underarm after bathing.

- Use pads for protection during your period. If using cloth, wash daily.

- Wipe private parts from *front* to *back* with toilet paper after using the toilet.

- Wash hands with soap and water after using the toilet and after changing sanitary napkins.

- Change underwear daily.

- Change your pads or tampons every three or four hours, or as often as necessary. This will keep you comfortable and help you to prevent odor from forming. If using tampons, make sure you change it every 4 to 8 hours. Longer tampon use can be dangerous to your health.

- Wrap disposable pads and tampons in toilet paper or paper and place them in the trash can for proper disposal. If using cloth pads, store the used pad in a sealable plastic bag and conceal it in your purse until you return home to rinse it out and wash it. Do not rinse reusable pads in public restrooms.

Your perineum area is sensitive. Vaginal washes should be researched before using. Douches, vaginal steaming, bubble baths, and bath bombs all have components or chemicals in them that will change your own body's natural pH balance. Women may find that they are sensitive to products and it could increase vaginal infections like overgrowth of unwanted bacteria.

Clothing (SW-p75)

Remaining in a wet bathing suit after swimming will also contribute to bacteria growth in the vaginal area. Towels should not be shared because they can pass along bacteria to other women.

Taking these precautions can help lower the risk of infection and keep the genitals healthy. Another part of good hygiene is being aware of what kind of clothes to wear and making sure that anything that touches the vaginal area is clean. A girl should wear cotton underwear or at least a pair with a cotton crotch. Underwear should be changed daily and after it becomes soiled or wet. It should be absorbent and well ventilated (cotton material is good for ventilation).

Tight or nylon underwear, tight pants, or pantyhose cause greater perspiration, which can allow bacteria to grow. (Note that most pantyhose brands are available with a cotton crotch, which helps ventilation.)

Deodorants vs. Antiperspirants

Another issue previously mentioned earlier in the course was body odor. But it's important to remember that, as you mature and go through puberty, your body odor changes and increases. Deodorants and antiperspirants come in many brands and varieties. Deodorants work to cover up body odor, while antiperspirants work to control, or dry up, perspiration. Our bodies are made to perspire, so if using a combination, be aware that you body needs to sweat. That is healthy for your body.

Many products now contain both a deodorant and an antiperspirant. These products come as aerosol sprays, roll-ons, sticks, creams, and even crystals. Choose the product that works right for you.

Just like with shaving, this is a topic that parents want to discuss in detail with their daughter when they feel she is ready for wearing this type of product.

Basic Skin Care

Taking good care of the skin involves a few basic steps. Dermatologists recommend that a person wash the face two times a day with a mild soap or gentle cleanser. It is best to avoid washing too often, as the skin will become irritated and dry out. If too much of the skin's natural oil is washed away, the skin may become very dry and begin to itch and flake. Because the skin's natural process is interrupted, the skin may begin to produce more oil than usual, which can cause more breakouts.

Dermatologists also recommend the following for clean, healthy skin:

- Use lotions only if needed and use ones that are oil-free and water-based.

- Try to identify what irritates the skin; if it's stress, try to reduce stress levels.

- Leave pimples alone. Picking, popping, or squeezing them will only make them worse. Have a dermatologist remove or extract pimples.

- Try to avoid touching the face. Also, regularly clean things that touch your face, like your phone, pillowcases, towel, etc.

- Antibacterial soaps are found to be harmful long term if using on regular basis, washing away the good bacteria as well as the bad.

- Keep hands clean by washing them often.

- Try to stay out of the sun, and use a sunscreen every day, year-round—even in the winter.

Other skin related items you might want to discuss with your students is the type of make up or nail polishes available that are more natural and not as chemically packed. For nail polish, when researching cleaner options, this doctor explains the two routes of absorption of the chemicals in nail polish:

"There are two routes of potential absorption: The nail plate (composed of densely packed keratin) or the surrounding nail folds and cuticle. Theoretically, absorption risk would be highest when in contact with the soft tissue (cuticle and nail folds) and would need to occur pre hardening of the lacquer. The other scenario would be nail biters who bite and ingest the cured polish," explains Dana Stern, M.D., a dermatologist with practices in New York City and Southampton, New York (https://www.womenshealthmag.com/beauty/g22665460/best-natural-nail-polishes/)

Considering your skin care and the makeup you use, we also have to seek out more healthy options for our skin. In the article, The Ultimate Guide to Clean Beauty, it states:

Clean beauty is a spectrum, but a case can be made that some ingredients should be avoided altogether. Below, the most common beauty ingredients of concern and the reasons why they're so notorious.

PARABENS | FRAGRANCES | ALUMINUM COMPOUNDS | ETHOXYLATED AGENTS | FORMALDEHYDE | REFINED PETROLEUM | HYDROQUINONE | TALC | TRICLOSAN | SILICA | OXYBENZONE

Skin Changes (SW-p-76)
Skin changes can be expected during adolescence. The onset of puberty means more hormones are produced by the body. It is these hormones that trigger the oil glands in the body's hair follicles to release more *sebum*, an oily substance made of fats, which may clog the small openings in the skin, called pores. With more sebum being produced, it is possible for the follicles to become clogged because the oil can't escape from the pore fast enough to make room for new sebum. If sebum and dead cells collect in the hair follicle, a white-colored plug will form in the pore. When this clogged pore gets irritated, it will swell and become red, creating a pimple.

Blackheads are also clogged pores, only darkened from oxidation. (Did you know that over the course of an average lifetime, a person will shed about 40 pounds of skin?)

Chapter 10
CELEBRATING OUR CYCLE

REVIEW (SW-p77)

- What are some warning signs that would indicate your cycle is not normal?
- What should you do if you cycle is not normal?

Celebrating & Preparing

There are many ways you can mark this momentous event in your life as a woman—and in this section we will talk about a few of those. How you celebrate is up to you!

- Purchase some needed items with your mother either online or at your favorite shops.
- Purchase a journal for special days to reflect and process all of the bodily changes.
- Write a letter to your mom with questions you may have or how she can help you during this time.
- Go way for the weekend with your mother and women family members to discuss your first cycle.
- Have a tea party with close friends, using nourishing herbal tea.
- Take a special bath or doing a spa day to acknowledge the changes.
- Get your ears pierced (with your mother's permission).
- Get a new purse or backpack to help ensure you have ample space for products for your period.

Quotes for Celebrating

Have the mothers take turns reading these quotes. Then, challenge the moms or daughters to come up with their own quote and share it with the rest of the class.

"Listen to and love your body, and learn to hit the pause button on purpose, rather than only when symptoms force you to." - Aviva Romm

"Approaching womanhood is an exciting time full of many new discoveries. It marks the beginning of a new era in your life where you get to be dependant on and solely trust the Lord for all things, including cycle health and wellness." - Doran Richards

"Menarche is a time of celebrating and acknowledging the beautiful process that God has allowed us to experience each cycle. Once we celebrate, embrace, and begin to understand our cycle, we can see that it is not a curse, but a perfect design." - Amy Hollon

"Women are awesome not because we can do the same things men can do but because we were made to do things that men can't do! We were designed in a way that every little thing about our bodies works together to produce LIFE. We are all here living this beautiful life because God designed our bodies to develop, grow, and nourish mankind!" - Ashley Spelllman

Celebrating with Blessingways

There is an event you can use to celebrate "coming of age" for young women called a blessingway.

"Rituals are society's way of teaching and maintaining the culture. To restore the matrilineal lines of initiation (old women teaching young women) rituals are essential. A menarche (first menstruation) ritual can make this time easier and more meaningful for both the young woman beginning menstruation, and her mother. Such a ritual comforts the young woman and lets her know that her feelings are natural and have been shared by women throughout time. It focuses the attention of the community on the young women's needs at this time in her life. And it instructs the young woman about what her family and society expect of her now that she is entering womanhood."

(Source:http://matriarchy.info/index.php?option=com_content&task=view&id=117)

The word ritual can sometimes be taken in context with rituals that are not God-honoring and of a wicked nature. But the word ritual simply means something done through generations and handed down and performed to mark an occasion.

When we perform the ritual of a blessingway for our daughters, we are creating a generational way of celebrating God's design for their body and for the bodies of the women to come. Blessingways can take many shapes, forms and sizes. It can be personal, small, and intimate or large, open and public. That is up to the individuals and to the mothers/guardians hosting such an event.

Step by step instructions can be found in the Appendix of this Teacher's Guide.

Closing Craft: Lapbooks

Wrapping up our wonderful time together, we want to go over some review questions and see if you know some things about your body and how it was created to function through menstruation.

Lapbooks & Memory Book Craft

We have finally gotten to a point in our class where we are going to start our craft! You get to take home a wonderful memory book, with what you have learned, to help you remember how your body is created to function.

We have cut outs and other prepared materials ready for you to glue into your blank books or lapbook folder design. You can add whatever you like to enhance the design and details. Some girls enjoy having other girls sign their books, as a reminder of who was with them during the workshop.

Benefits of Using Lapbooks

Welcome to the wonderful world of lapbooking. Lapbooking has become particularly popular with parents who have chosen to homeschool their children because you can get a whole lot of information crammed into one of them. There a several benefits of using lapbooks, whether you are educating your children at home or you just want some extra activities for your child to do. Let's take a look:

Lapbooks are a great way for children to review and help remember the information you are teaching them or that they are learning at school. They encourage your children to find the information they are looking for instead of having it handed to them. Studies have also proven that, when children are given hands-on activities to learn while they study, they will retain more information.

Lapbooks are a great way for children and students to keep a close eye on what they are learning. With a lapbook, you can keep track of the major concepts you learn with each unit or theme (depending on how you make them) and your child can see the progress they are making and how much they have learned. This will help them stay motivated to keep working on their projects.

Possibilities are endless when it comes to making lapbooks. You don't have to homeschool to make one of these books for your children. They are a learning tool to use with education or just increase knowledge while doing something fun with your children. If your child loves trains, then make a lapbook about trains; if they love insects then try making one about insects.

Lapbooks are extremely developmentally appropriate for all different ages and all different learning styles. Lapbooks can be custom made to meet the needs of a child with a learning disability or a child that is exceptionally bright and gifted in a certain area.

Creating a lapbook helps children learn many different skills that they will need. Younger children can learn how to cut and paste pictures, do a little research, and even some sequencing. For older children, they can learn how to do some serious research, gain some computer skills, take notes, and learn some important writing skills. Children can also learn how to organize their work in an orderly manner and how to present the material in a good way.

Most important, perhaps, is the fact that they are making something that they can take pride in and they will use. Lapbooks aren't just something you make and feel like you don't need or can just throw into the trash can like some of the other educational things students bring home. They can really increase their knowledge and help them improve some important skills. They can really feel like they're spending time producing something that is worthwhile and worth keeping.

Evaluation Forms

The evaluation form is a great tool to be better teaching the workshop each time. Invite them to take part in the evaluation, provided in the **Appendix** and on the website **blessingsgodsway.com**, and turn it in before they leave.

NOTE: Ask the mothers:

Please take a few minutes to fill this evaluation form out completely and hand in to the instructor before leaving. We ask that you give constructive criticism as well as what has blessed you throughout the learning process of this curriculum. The information is used to make the course better for others. I thank you in advance for this time and effort to fill it out.

Certificates of Completion

Hand each daughter a certificate of completion. You can make your own or use the one provided in the **Appendix** of this Teacher's Guide. We have also provided a PDF version you can download from the Blessings God's Way website **www.BlessingGodsWay.com**

NOTE: Inform the parents:

Please keep these certificates as keepsakes from our day together. This was an intensive course and you did it! My prayer is that it will enable you to see your body's design as a blessing to you, God's way. Also, that you would grow up and take this information and teach it to the next generation, your daughters. "Each one, teach one" is a great philosophy.

APPENDICES

Appendix 1
MAIDENHOOD COURSE QUIZZES

You can choose to do one quiz or all three with your students.

That will depend on time and how long you want to spend doing review.

Please find each individual quiz on the following pages.

QUIZ #1

Please fill in the answers:

What does the word menses mean?

What is the name of my body part that sheds a lining each month once menses begins?

What are two physical changes that take place in my body when I go through puberty?

The egg, once released from the ovary, passes through my ________________ tube.

What are two ways I can take my thoughts captive during menstruation?

I have two hormones that need to stay in balance called:

The talk about blood should not be fearful or scary because:

When I menstruate, there are other elements to the liquid that my body is disposing of, one of them being?

What can I do during menstruation to help me relax, rest and be Christ-like in all I do?

I can celebrate menstruation many different ways, one of them being:

What does the culture tell you about your cycle that you know is not true according to God's design?

How can you combat a spirit of fear surrounding this season in your life?

Should you discuss this issue with mere acquaintances? Yes or No?

QUIZ #2

The Female Reproductive System - Side Body View

Please label each blank line:

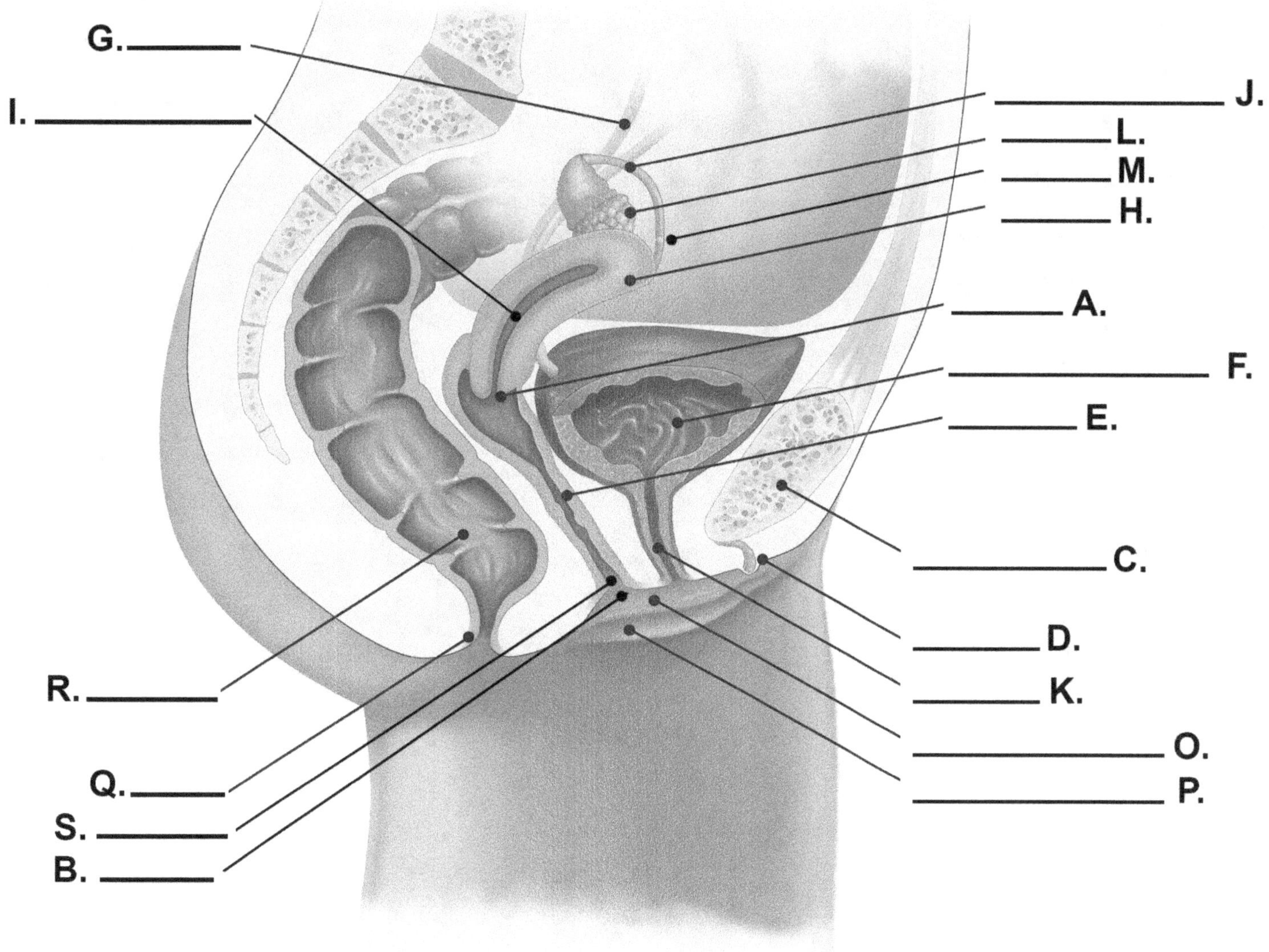

QUIZ #3

The Female Reproductive System - Front View

Please label each blank line:

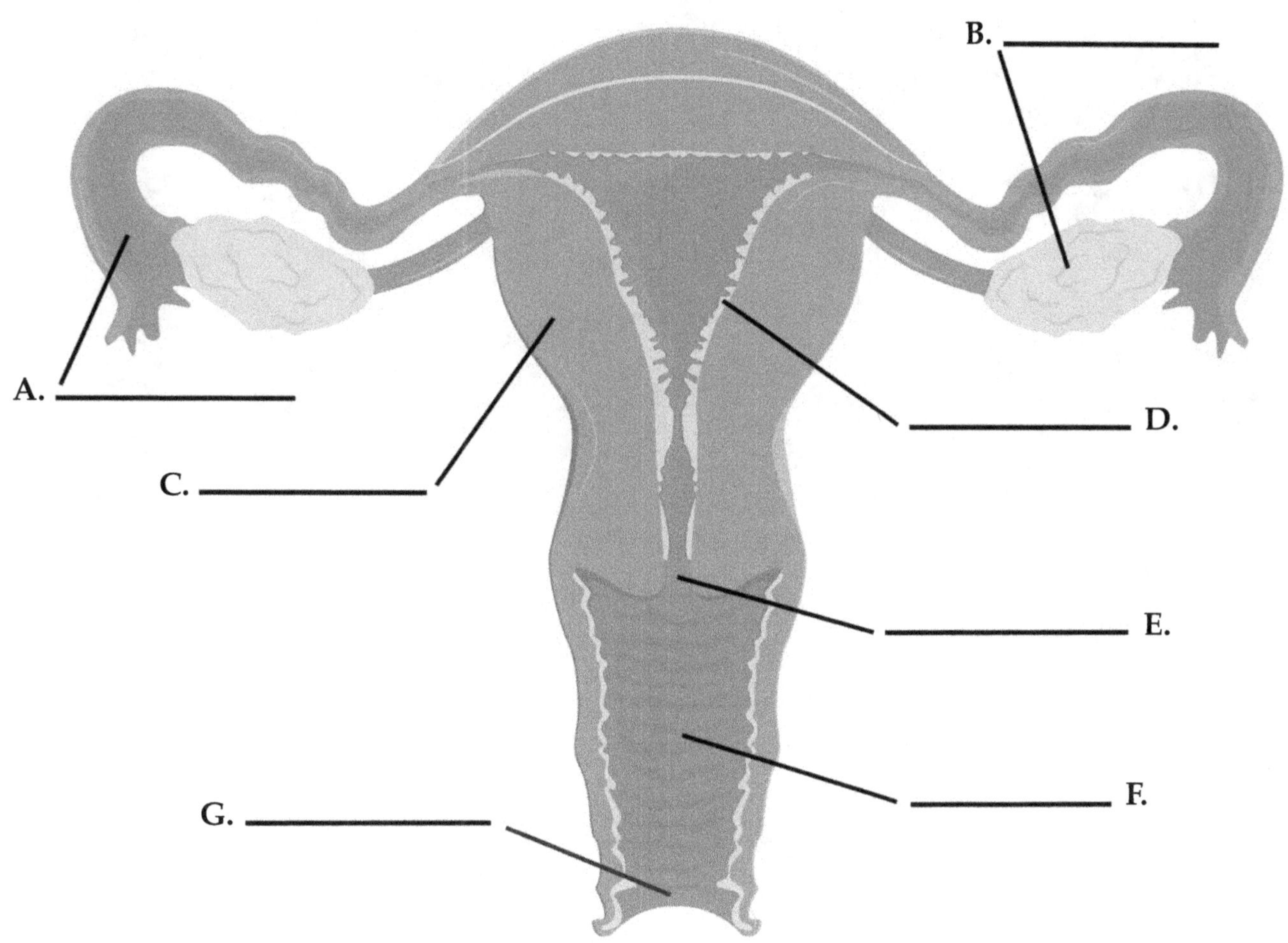

Appendix 2
FORMS

Evaluation Form

Certificate of Achievement

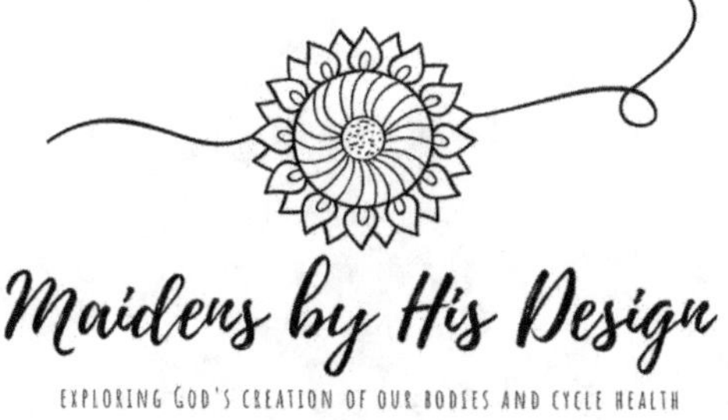

Evaluation Form

Name: ____ Date: _______________

What are 3 facts you have learned by taking this course?

Would you recommend this course to other women and daughters?

Do you believe your knowledge has increased for understanding the way God has created your body and how it functions?

Would you share with us constructive criticism for how we can better teach this curriculum?

Would you give us a word of testimony for your experience that we can use as testimony when promoting this material in social media and on the website?

Any last questions or comments?

Certificate of Achievement

This Certifies that

____

*Has successfully completed the training
program requirement for*

Maidens by His Design

EXPLORING GOD'S CREATION OF OUR BODIES AND OUR CYCLE HEALTH.

___________________   ___________________
DATE   MOTHER/AUNT/GRANDMA

Appendix 3
CELEBRATING WITH A BLESSINGWAY

I am placing here a step-by-step section for you to use next time you have an opportunity to serve a friend or family member by celebrating the onset of their first cycle beginning, the gift of their child, or the waning of their cycle. When a young woman begins her cycle, consider having a few very close friends over with their mothers and have a special gathering teaching them to see God in their lives for this season. For maternity, you can celebrate the new life for this family and give her encouragement and inspiration to see God's honor bestowed upon her in the gift of their child. When a woman reaches menopause, life has shifted and moved in a different direction. That change can be acknowledged and honored for her. A Blessingway is a great opportunity to recognize the changes, supporting her through the transition that sometimes can be very drastic or span over a few years.

Our culture has misguided pictures of what these seasons are supposed to be in our lives. Celebrating with a Blessingway gathering provides us with a way to be a good example; shedding a light into the darkness that is often so prevalent. Having a Blessingway allows the hostess to exercise her gifts of hospitality and service towards others. It allows the guest of honor to take time out of her busy life, as well as providing a time of joy and fellowship to the guests and the one who is hosting.

Why celebrate? First and foremost, we want to give honor, glory and praise to our God for His gift of whichever cycle or phase we are in. Secondly, we want to bring women and families together to celebrate and give support to the honored guest in their new season of life.

The word blessing means "a short prayer for divine approval." To bless a young woman experiencing her first cycle, we are invoking God's favor upon her for her "way," the journey, and through her transition ahead. Women need support and encouragement throughout their seasons and having a Blessingway provides this through scripture reading, praise to our LORD, singing of songs, and partaking in a meal together.

Before continuing on, please remember that a Blessingway is an avenue for women and families to come together to give honor to God for either the onset of menstruation for their daughter or loved one, for the gift of a child, or for the blessing of menopause when our cycle ceases to exist and we begin a new phase in life. By encouraging celebrations for pregnancy, we are not advocating any particular point of view in the area of family planning. Each of us has our own relationship with the LORD, and we walk out our paths differently. The Blessing God's Way ministry teaches a simpler message, that God is the Giver and Creator of menstruation, children, and our cycles ending, and that they all are a blessing.

Materials List

Below you will find a list of materials that we hope will be helpful in planning a Blessingway. Feel free to gather the materials yourself.

- Hairbrush
- Hair ties, pins
- Dried or real flowers
- Very warm water
- Basin for foot bath
- Lighter or matches
- Box of tissues
- Pillows
- Towel
- Soothing Music
- Invitations
- Games
- Sand for a tray of candles
- Candles for the tray of sand
- Herbs for foot wash
- Massage Oil for Massage
- Tea light candles (or ask guests to bring them)
- This book for reproducible materials and resources to share
- Beads to create necklaces or bracelets
- Henna powder (organic and from reputable source) for temporary tattoos
- Scripture cards (made or purchased)

Special Surroundings

We all have those favorite areas in our home where we can unwind and feel relaxed. For the Blessingway, we want to create that area for her, as well as adding an extra amount of comfort to the surroundings, if possible. The honored guest needs a place where she can see all the "pretties" around her, where she can feel joy and happiness by simply looking around the room. A suggestion would be to touch the five senses in some manner:

- Get out special cloths or spreads to stretch out on the ground where you will gather;

- Fill the room with fresh flowers from the outdoors;

- Have candles burning to create a light that is pleasing and welcoming;

- Depending on the weather, use the outdoors to have fresh air blowing and crisp air to breathe;

- Make sure all the chairs, spreads and pillows soft and smooth to the touch;

- Have spiritual and encouraging music playing softly in the background.

Fellowship Meal

At the closing of a Blessingway, the guests are asked to gather and partake in a meal together. Sharing fellowship with one another is part of this celebration. Always remember our food is from Him and of Him. We are being filled with the bread of life! One of the benefits of Jesus dying on the cross is that we can entertain and share a fellowship meal with our loved ones. Food is a blessing. It is also nourishing, sustaining and life giving.

"Bread is made for laughter..." **- Ecclesiastes 10:19**

"...But the cheerful of heart has a continual feast." **- Proverbs 15:15**

(For women having a baby or are going through menopause, you can use a food train sign up list to encourage meal trains for their time of transition. There are plenty of online resources to do this electronically as well.)

Additional Tips & Suggestions

Over the years I have gotten so many suggestions and tips for celebrating. I hope these are helpful as you put together your Blessingway gathering.

Breaking bread with one another in a fellowship meal is an intimate gesture. It should be sweet and lasting (not in a hurry to get everyone out and home when the clock strikes 2:00). We don't mean to say that you should keep everyone in your home all day, either, of course! Have a time schedule for the Blessingway, but don't be too harsh in sticking to the minute of it. Remember, we want to make a statement of "relax" to our honored guest and friends.

A Blessingway is an intimate gathering for close friends and loved ones. When you make your invitation list, make sure you include people who are comfortable around one another. Of course, everyone present does not have to be a Christian. We pray that by hearing the word of God at this gathering their hearts will be turned to Him. We know that scripture does not come back void!

When inviting women and young ladies to a Blessingway, consider inviting husbands and other children to take part in this celebration. In some instances, this would be appropriate, but in other instances it wouldn't. Remember this is a time for the honored guest to relax, and sometimes having little children around would defeat that purpose. The focus should be first on the LORD, then on the honored guest, and then on the rest of the family/friends present.

The host or another guest could start a scrapbook with all the poems, blessing and thoughts that were presented at the gathering. The honored guest would then have the scrapbook, which she may like to look at while she is in her time of month, in labor or going through menopause. This can be very encouraging to her. A Blessingway scrapbook paper album has been available for this occasion. This can be purchased from Blessing God's Way online, or you can purchase a plain one from your favorite store.

Taking and developing photos from the Blessingway would be an awesome addition to the scrapbook when completed. Having the photos to view will be a treat and joy for the honored guest and her family for years to come.

Some women enjoy making a prayer bracelet or necklace for the honored guest. You can do this by asking everyone to bring a bead and with it, they can give their "gift from the heart". The young lady, mother, or menopausal woman could wear this in remembrance of the women or ladies who stand behind her and who have gone before her.

Henna has become a popular way of expressing love and community, especially as a reassurance that you have a "tribe" who supports you in the season of life you are in. You can look into having henna designs done either on the guest of honor only (hand, belly, feet) or everyone can have a small design created. Be aware not to use cheap, black henna ink, which can cause side effects from the chemicals used. Instead, purchase organic henna powder from reputable resource.

If you are hosting this Blessingway for adopting parents or parents who have experienced loss, consider being more mindful and sensitive to the family you serve. Families who adopt have gone through a vigorous process to finally obtain official papers and custody, so we want to honor them for enduring that process and give God glory for it. For those who have had a loss, a Blessingway can be used to recognize that this mom was pregnant and there still is a baby to be celebrated. It is a tool to help a mom process the grief and share her story as she continues to heal.

I have quoted scripture on big paper and taped it to the walls in the room where the women will be meeting and celebrating. This is a reminder to hide His word in our heart, and the honored guest can take them home as a keepsake and re-tape them on their walls for extra help focusing on God's goodness to them. Affirmation Cards are also wonderful encouragement and reminders.

Basic Instructional Outline for a Blessingway
Choose either an indoor or outdoor special place to host the Blessingway. You will need the materials from the kit. Go out of your way to make the surroundings as inviting and pretty as you can.

Gather the group in a circle. At this time, you can introduce yourself and explain why you have chosen to do a Blessingway.

Offer up prayer to begin. You could offer thanks to our LORD for the person you are honoring and the transition she is about to go through, for God's goodness in His blessing to her in this phase of life, asking for guidance and strength for her upcoming cycle/s. You could pray over the time spent during the gathering, that it would bring glory to Him Who makes all things! (See the sample prayer below or make up your own.)

Sample prayer for opening a Blessingway:

We thank you LORD for this day, for this time to gather and give you glory for such a great gift as being a woman made by your perfect design. You have made us fearfully and wonderfully and we know that full well. We are grateful you have called us to come together to support, encourage and uplift this young lady/woman. Give us a humble and serving spirit toward this honored guest. Please bless our time and the people gathered here today. We pray this in Jesus Christ's name, Amen.

Now would be a good time to sing the Doxology, which is a wonderful opening song to give praise and thanks to the LORD. Again, you want to help all the participants to focus on the true reason for such a joyous occasion.

Praise God from Whom all blessings flow,

Praise Him all creatures here below,

Praise Him above ye heavenly host,

Praise Father, Son, and Holy Ghost

Have all participants introduce themselves and share how they know the honored guest. You could also implement another icebreaker to get everyone relaxed and comfortable.

Let's sing! Singing songs, giving praise and glory to our LORD, is an important part of this gathering.

Next, you can share how this gathering is meant to give glory to God for the particular cycle and encourage the honored guest by giving blessings from the heart and words of encouragement and support. You can speak of how God has designed our bodies for our cycles and that His grace is sufficient. Point out how 40 weeks (the time of gestation for pregnancy and the time a woman menstruates on average) is a number God uses over and over for transitions that bring about great change and blessing. The number 40 is often understood as the "number of probation or trial." For example, the Israelites wandered for 40 years (Deuteronomy 8:2-5); Moses was on the mount for 40 days (Exodus 24:18); 40 days were involved in the story of Jonah and Nineveh (Jonah 3:4); Jesus was tempted for 40 days (Matthew 4:2); there were 40 days between Jesus' resurrection and ascension (Acts 1:3). He describes to us that these times are for testing our hearts and minds, but that, in the end, the "promised land" is oh, so sweet to behold, making it all worthwhile!

"The whole commandment that I command you to- day you shall be careful to do, that you may live and multiply, and go in and possess the land that the LORD swore to give your fathers. And you shall remember the whole way that the LORD your God has led you these forty years in the wilderness, that He might humble you, testing you to know what was in your heart, whether you would keep His commandments or not... For the LORD your God is bringing you into a good land, a land of brooks of water, of fountains and springs, flowing out in the valleys and hills; ...and you shall bless the LORD your God for the good land which He has given you." **- Deuteronomy 8:1-10**

Decorate the honored guest's hair with flowers (fresh, dried, fabric, fake). Having the younger girls braid and brush her hair is very touching and they really enjoy this part. You could also make a crown of flowers, putting that on her when her hair is finished being brushed or braided.

Next you can get a bowl filled with warm/hot water and pour in the herbs with a few drops of massage oil (almond, coconut or olive oil is preferred). Make sure you have plenty of towels nearby. Let the honored guest soak her feet for a few minutes (a good time to sing or play a song). Have her mother wash her feet (if present), then the mother-in-law, sisters or best friends. Open it up to whoever would like to participate. Singing another song here would be nice. Talk about how this is an ultimate gesture of humility and service toward one another as it may be uncomfortable for both. Nonetheless, it is a spiritual experience you will not forget easily. Most women who are unsure about this portion usually exclaim how wonderful it was to do or to have it done to them. It brings a feeling of vulnerability, but one of complete servanthood as well.

> "If I then, your Lord and Teacher, have washed your feet, you also ought to wash one another's feet." **- John 13:14**

Massage the feet with the foot massage oil. Ask for others to come and help. You might also want to massage her hands, just to give the honored guest a little extra pampering. Massage is medicinal, moving circulation in the body and reducing swelling and aches.

> "Oil and perfume make the heart glad." **- Proverbs 27:9**

Now is the time to light candles. Share any special handmade gifts, poems, blessings, or thoughts for encouragement. The lighting of candles is simply used to remind us that the LORD is our Light and gives us light. One person lights her candle and gives her gift from the heart, then the next person in the circle does the same. A gift from the heart can be a drawing, scripture or anything that comes from the heart with meaning and love.

> "The LORD is my light and my salvation; whom shall I fear? The LORD is the stronghold of my life; of whom shall I be afraid?" **- Psalm 27:1**

Explain to the honored guest the she can re-light these candles when she starts her period that month, goes into labor or when she is having a very bad menopause day. She then can be reminded of all those gathered at the Blessingway and how they are supporting her in spirit.

Have the first person light a candle, place it in the tray, then present their words and/or blessing, advice or drawing (gift from the heart). The next person lights candle and does the same. Continue all the way around the circle.

Once all the prayers, blessings, and poems are gathered, give them to the honored guest with a scrapbook for her to make a keepsake. Or, as suggested previously, give a scrapbook and contents to the guest who volunteered to compile it.

> "In all things I have shown that by working hard in this way we must help the weak and remember the words of the LORD Jesus, how he himself said, "It is more blessed to give than to receive." **- Acts 20:35**

> "For you were called to freedom, brothers. Only do not use your freedom as an opportunity for the flesh, but through love serve one another. For the whole law is fulfilled in one word: 'You shall love your neighbor as yourself.'" - **Galatians 5:13-14**

Now would be a good time to present the gift certificate if you have compiled contributions for this. A gift card or certificate would be useful to treat herself or to save for a rainy day. For an expecting mother, it can be used to get exactly what she needs for that particular pregnancy.

Finally, pray again, laying hands on the honored woman, asking a blessing on the food you are about to partake and for a blessing upon the honored guest. Invite everyone to stay and eat and be merry!

> "And I commend joy, for man has nothing better under the sun but to eat and drink and be joyful, for this will go with him in his toil through the days of his life that God has given him under the sun." - **Ecclesiastes 8:15**

Introduce the concept of a Food Train Sign Up for bringing meals to a woman after having her baby or for a woman dealing with difficult menopause symptoms or for a young lady to spark some light in their lives & uplift them with food that they enjoy! Only the pregnancy sign up would require a week's worth of meals... the other cycles and phases of womanhood could use maybe one a month or when appropriate.

WORKS CITED

Abdallah, Amy F. Davis. "How I Learned to Love My Period". *Christianity Today*.http://www.christianitytoday.com/women/2016/march/how-i-learned-to-love-my-period.html

Bell, James S. Jr., Ed. Gliksman, Michele Isaacs. DiGeronimo, Theresa Foy. Lee, Janet. *The Christian Family Guide to Pregnancy and Childbirth*. Penguin Group, 2013

Bennet, Jane. *A Blessing Not a Curse: A Mother-Daughter Guide to the Transition from Girl to Woman*. Sally Milner Publishing Pty Ltd, 2002.

Bennett, Robin Rose. *The Gift of Healing Herbs: Plant Medicines and Home Remedies for a Vibrantly Healthy Life*. North Atlantic Books. 2014.

Bhartiya, Aru. "Menstruation, Religion and Society." *International Journal of Social Science and Humanity*. Vol. 3, No. 6. November 2013.

Bremness, Lesley. *Principles & Practice of Phytotherapy: Modern Herbal Medicine, 2nd Ed*. Churchill Livingston, 2013.

DiStasio, Joan. *Biology*. 1995. Frank Schaffer Publications, School House Publishing.

Freda, Daniela. "Four Signs of a Healthy Menstrual Cycle that Every Woman Should Know." https://danielafreda.com/2013/09/24/four-signs-of-a-healthy-menstrual-cycle-that-all-women-should-know/

Ganz, Richard L. "Six Ways to Take Your Thoughts Captive."

http://www.crosswalk.com/faith/prayer/prayers/take-your-thoughts-captive-509888.html

"Getting Rid of Body Hair: For Young Teens." Women's and Children's Health Network. www.cyh.com/HealthTopics/HealthTopicDetailsKids.aspx?p=335&np=289&id=2407

Goldbeck, Nikki. As You Eat So Your Baby Grows: A Guide to Nutrition in Pregnancy. Ceres Press, 2000.

Hale, Mabel. *Beautiful Girlhood*. Brownstone Books, 2009.

Hoffman, David. *The Herbal Handbook: A User's Guide to Medical Herbalism*. Healing Arts, 1998.

Hoffman, David. *The New Holistic Herbal*. Element Books, Ltd, 1991.

Hoffman, David. *Medical Herbalism: The Science and Practice of Herbal Medicine*. Healing Arts, 2003.

"Massage During Menstruation." Massage Envy Franchising, LLC., 2018.

https://www.massageenvy.com/massage/massage-benefits/massage-during-menstruation/

Mayo Clinic Staff. "Toxic Shock Syndrome." Mayo Foundation for Medical Education and Research. https://www.mayoclinic.org/diseases-conditions/toxic-shock-syndrome/symptoms-causes/syc-20355384

McDaniel, Debbie. "33 Verses to Remind us We Do Not have to Fear." http://www.crosswalk.com/blogs/debbie-mcdaniel/33-verses-to-remind-us—we-do-not-have-to-fear.html

McIntyre, Anne. *The Complete Woman's Herbal: A Manual of Healing Herbs and Nutrition for Personal Well-Being and Family Care*. Holt Paperbacks, 1995.

O'Donnell, Jennifer and Richard N. Fogoros, MD."Shaving Tips for Preteen Girls: What's the Right Age for a Girl to Start Shaving. http://parentingteens.about.com/cs/familylife/a/girlsshaving.htm

Pederson, Mark. *Nutritional Herbology: A Reference Guide to Herbs*. Whitman Pubns, 1998.

"Puberty." American Academy of Pediatrics. www.aap.org/family/puberty.htm

Queen, Sandi. *From Girl…To Woman*. www.queenhomeschool.com

Romm, Aviva. "The Top Daily Supplements for Women."https://avivaromm.com/nutritional-supplements- for-women/

Stang, Jamie and Mary Story."Adolescent Growth and Development." *Guidelines for Adolescent Nutrition Services*. Center for Leadership, Education and Training in Maternal and Child Nutrition: Minnesota, 2005

"The Facts on Tampons--And How to Use Them Safely." US Department of Health and Human Services, 2018. https://www.fda.gov/ForConsumers/ConsumerUpdates/ucm612029.htm

Trobisch, Ingrid. *The Joy of Being a Woman*. San Francisco, California: Harper San Francisco, 1980, 1980.

"TSS." Menstruation.com. https://www.menstruation.com.au/periodpages/tss.html

"Using Your First Tampon." Center for Young Women's Health. 2016. https://youngwomenshealth.org/2012/09/27/tampons/

Weed, Susus S. *Wise Woman Herbal for the Childbearing Year*. Informed Homebirth, 1986.

"What We Believe" Holy Yoga. Holy Yoga Global LLC, 2017. https://holyyoga.net/about/what-we-believe/

Wood, Matthew. *The Book of Herbal Wisdom: Using Plants for Medicine.* North Atlantic Books. 2017.

Wood, Matthew. *The Earthwise Herbal Volume I: A Complete Guide to Old World Medicinal Plants.* North Atlantic Books, 2011.

Wood, Matthew. *The Earthwise Herbal Volume II: A Complete Guide to Old World Medicinal Plants.* North Atlantic Books, 2011.

Zenack, Marie. "First Menstruation Ritual." Understanding the Nonviolent Society: Matriarchy. 2000-2007. http://matriarchy.info/index.php?option=com_content&task=view&id=117

www.ingramcontent.com/pod-product-compliance
Lightning Source LLC
Chambersburg PA
CBHW081618250726
48657CB00009B/2609